Speech and Language Intervention in Down Syndrome

Edited by

Jean A. Rondal PhD
University of Liège, Belgium

and

Sue Buckley BA, CPsychol
University of Portsmouth, UK

W

Whurr Publishers Ltd
London

© 2003 Whurr Publishers Ltd
First published 2003
by Whurr Publishers Ltd
19b Compton Terrace
London N1 2UN
England

Reprinted 2004

British Library Cataloguing in Publication Data
A catalogue record for this book is available from the British Library.

ISBN 1 86156 296 9

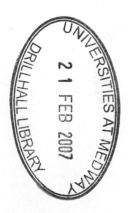

Typeset by Adrian McLaughlin, a@microguides.net
Printed and bound by Antony Rowe Ltd, Eastbourne

Contents

Preface

From the 'idiocy of the Mongolian type' (Down, 1866), or the 'Kalmuk idiocy' (Frazer and Mitchell, 1876), the Langdon Down syndrome, or perhaps more historically accurately the Seguin-Down syndrome (Stratford, 1999) has come a long way to the present time. The French physician Edouard Seguin, first President of the American Association on Mental Deficiency after his departure from France, appears to have been the first author to allude (at least) to the condition; cf. Seguin (1846). In 1959, Lejeune and his collaborators identified that 'mongolism' was etiologically related to trisomy 21 (Lejeune, Gautier and Turpin, 1959a, b). The birth of a child with Down syndrome is no longer associated with atavistic regression, parental sin, alcoholism, congenital syphilis, maternal tuberculosis, or even bad thinking during pregnancy. Average life expectancy has increased tremendously from a few years at the turn of the twentieth century to more than 50 years in the 1980s (Baird and Sadovnik, 1988) – probably more as of today – and perhaps to increase yet in the coming decades.

In the same way, we have long bypassed Esquirol's negative pronouncements concerning the treatment of 'idiocy'. Esquirol (1838), often regarded as the father of modern psychiatry, professed that it was useless to try to treat idiocy because it would amount to changing the structure of the brain and this was (and still is) beyond reach. However, from 1840 the young Seguin (inspired by Itard's attempt at civilizing the 'wild boy of Aveyron') defied Esquirol's prediction and set about educating 'mentally handicapped' children in his hospital.

We have come a long way since the times when children with Down syndrome were classed as ineducable or, at best, thought of as rarely educable. Now the typical expectation is that the majority of these children, if properly educated, will learn to develop acceptable levels of independence. Promising future developments are probably linked with the move towards more school and social inclusion.

The present work is the heir to this difficult but meritorious past. It incorporates the reasonable belief that in a domain such as language, which currently benefits from an extensive accumulation of knowledge, it should be possible to increase significantly the effectiveness of the intervention strategies and programmes in such a way as to largely compensate for the problems typical of the condition of Down syndrome.

Jean A Rondal

References

Baird P, Sadovnik A (1988) Life expectancy in Down's syndrome adults. Lancet 1354–6.

Down JL (1866) Observations on an ethnic classification of idiots. Hospital Clinical Lectures and Reports 3: 259.

Esquirol J (1838) Des Maladies Mentales (2 volumes). Paris: Baillière.

Frazer J, Mitchell A (1876) Report on a case with autopsy and notes on 62 cases. Journal of Mental Science 22: 169–72.

Lejeune J, Gautier M, Turpin R (1959a) Les chromosomes humains en culture de tissus. Comptes-rendus Hebdomadaires des Séances de l'Académie des Sciences 248: 602–3.

Lejeune J, Gautier M, Turpin R (1959b) Etude des chromosomes somatiques de neuf enfants mongoliens. Comptes-rendus Hebdomadaires des Séances de l'Académie des Sciences 248: 1721–2.

Seguin E (1846) Idiocy: Its Treatment by the Physiological Method. New York: Wood.

Stratford B (1999) Down syndrome: treatment and attitudes in the past, at present and in the future. Journal of Pediatrics, Obstetrics and Gynaecology (November/December): 9–16, 34.

Contributors

Leonard Abbeduto PhD, Professor of Educational Psychology and Associate Director for Behavioral Sciences, Waisman Center, University of Wisconsin-Madison, USA

Angela M Becerra BA, Graduate student, Department of Psychological and Brain Sciences, University of Louisville, USA

Sue Buckley BA, CPsychol. Emeritus Professor, Department of Psychology, University of Portsmouth and Director of Research, The Down Syndrome Educational Trust, Portsmouth, UK

John Clibbens PhD, Reader, Department of Psychology, University of Plymouth, UK

Frances A Conners PhD, Associate Professor of Psychology, University of Alabama, USA

Yolanda Keller-Bell PhD, Postdoctoral Fellow, Waisman Center, University of Wisconsin-Madison, USA

Christine Jenkins PhD, Senior lecturer, Department of Psychology, University of Portsmouth, UK

Carolyn B Mervis, Distinguished University Scholar and Professor, Department of Psychological and Brain Sciences, University of Louisville, USA

Carol Stoel-Gammon PhD, Professor of Speech and Hearing Sciences, University of Washington, Seattle, USA

Gaye Powell MRCSLT, PhD, Research Associate, Human Communication Studies, The College of St Mark and St John Plymouth, and Associate Member: Centre for Thinking and Language, Department of Psychology, University of Plymouth, UK

Jean A Rondal PhD, Dr Linguistique et Sciences du Langage. Professeur Ordinaire (full professor) de Psychologie et de Psycholinguistique, Département des Sciences Cognitives, Université de Liège, Belgium

Chapter 1
Principles of language intervention

JEAN A RONDAL, SUE BUCKLEY

Principles

The descriptive and experimental study of speech, language and communication development and functioning in Down syndrome, which has
made important progress particularly since the mid-1970s, should now
give more attention to the definition and justification of approaches and
strategies for intervention (rehabilitation or remediation). In our view,
language intervention with individuals with Down syndrome should be
based on sound principles and take account of the set of interrelated
dimensions illustrated in Figure 1.1.

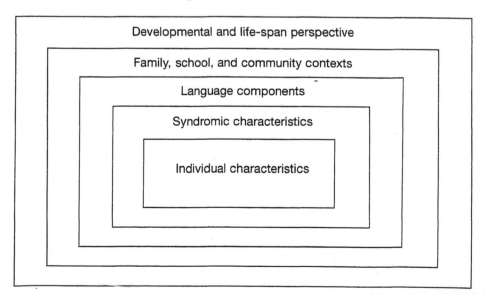

Figure 1.1. Major dimensions of language intervention with Down syndrome
persons.

1

Intervention must be developmental in the sense of the term used by Rondal and Edwards (1997) and (more generally – in other words, outside the language domain) of Cicchetti and Beeghly (1990). Research increasingly shows that development and functioning in individuals with intellectual disabilities are as organized, purposeful, and adaptive as in typically developing individuals, albeit with limitations and difficulties. From this perspective the quantitative and qualitative differences between typically developing individuals and individuals with intellectual disabilities are viewed as variations in basically similar processes or as pathological distortions of otherwise normal phases of development.

Numerous observations (cf. Rosenberg and Abbeduto, 1993; Rondal and Edwards, 1997 for systematic reviews) suggest that language development in individuals with intellectual disabilities, including those with Down syndrome, proceeds, in major ways, as it does in typically developing individuals. Similar sequences of steps are documented until final plateaux are reached. Development in individuals with intellectual disabilities is slower and remains incomplete in many respects. There are no clear indications, however, that the basic mechanisms involved in each domain of language development radically differ. This suggests that intervention programmes should follow typical development as closely as possible. More specifically, programmes that closely follow the indications on the sequences of development within the various language components are likely to be more effective. Graduated sequences of training for prelinguistic, cognitive-semantic, phonological, lexical, morphosyntactic, pragmatic, and discursive skills, can be implemented with children and adolescents with Down syndrome. The general objective of the intervention programmes can be summarized as follows: 'to enable persons with Down syndrome to master as quickly and as completely as possible the sequences of skills characteristic of normal development'. It is believed that early and continued intervention, when conducted adequately, carries the best chances of reducing further disabilities, given the cumulative nature of the developmental process.

Language intervention should be age related. Language difficulties and obstacles vary considerably from the baby to the ageing person with Down syndrome. Age-appropriate intervention can and should be implemented.

The present book begins with the prelinguistic stages and discusses intervention principles applicable to babies and infants that encourage an earlier emergence of language than would be the case otherwise, and continues by examining remedial measures and measures to enhance language activities for children, adolescents and young adults, and language maintenance in ageing persons with Down syndrome.

Quite clearly, language development is a dynamic, interactive, and social process as well as an individual, brain-based, and cognitively dependent process; therefore families, schools, and communities matter considerably in any intervention perspective. In fact, early intervention cannot be effective outside of the family setting and without the active participation of the parents or caretakers of the child with Down syndrome. Schools and communities ought to be more closely associated with the remediation intervention perspective in intellectual disabilities, and Down syndrome in particular. Whatever the merits of a given intervention strategy, it will have only a limited effect in furthering development and functioning if the attitudes and opportunities of the inclusive educational or community setting are less than appropriate. This, of course, should come as no surprise. We do not develop skills, whether physical, cognitive, linguistic, or social, just for the sake of private personal satisfaction, but rather, at least partially, for use in social settings and with socio-functional aims.

Language organization is basically (but not exclusively) modular, meaning that language is not, despite appearances, a unitary phenomenon. It results from the appropriate integration of various components (such as phonological, lexical, morphosyntactic, pragmatic, and discursive aspects) which are autonomous to a large extent, as numerous pathological observations indicate. The specificity of these major language components is such that attempts to implement multipurpose remediation procedures are bound to generate only mediocre effects. The modularity perspective is central to the organization of this book, as can be seen from an inspection of the table of contents. Individual chapters relate to the various components of the language system. One chapter also deals with memory training, and more particularly with phonological or auditory/verbal working memory. Several aspects and components of the language system may crucially depend on the integrity or, at least, the minimal effectiveness of the short-term memory systems, allowing the temporary storage and processing of information, alongside information retrieved from longer-term memories. Children with Down syndrome seem to have particular weaknesses in these aspects of cognitive development and functioning. It is therefore important to include activities aimed at improving working memory in individuals with Down syndrome in order to set the stage for better language and cognitive development.

The diverse modalities of language functioning also need to be taken into account. Spoken language, of course, is of utmost importance. It raises the problem of the particular speech difficulties that are common in individuals with Down syndrome. There is no good reason, as will be argued in more detail later in the book, to exclude children with Down syndrome from written language learning and literacy training, as was generally the case even in the recent past. The idea that children with Down syndrome can achieve functional levels of literacy, when properly taught, is gradually gaining ground. Moreover, it is becoming clear that reading and writing may be beneficial for overall language acquisition. This may be particularly true for children with Down syndrome who have better visual perceptual and visual memory abilities than auditory ones.

Language can also be developed using nonverbal systems of communication. A number of such systems are available: from manual sign languages, such as the American or the British sign language, mainly used by deaf people, or simplified versions of these, to numerous visual systems relying on pictographic logographs and multimodality approaches. The potential benefits of the different systems have to be evaluated for each individual. Alternative and augmentative systems of communication (AASC) may have a role in facilitating effective communication in people with intellectual disabilities. They can create a pathway to speech, setting improved communication contexts for better interpretation and more accurate use of the sounds of spoken language. In children whose spoken language is seriously delayed, they can complement the speech that these subjects have already learned or are learning. Alternative and augmentative systems of communication can also provide a substitute for speech in individuals with little possibility of acquiring vocal fluency for organic reasons. For this reason, and with regard to the communication difficulties of profoundly deaf people, it would be a good idea if those in charge of administering the schools in our countries would recommend teaching and learning sign language as a second or third language from the early ages for all children. Expressing oneself in a 'space language' is great fun. The children would enjoy it. It could be cognitively fruitful in promoting a sort of linguistic 'decentration' by exposing the children to a three-dimensional language system in addition to the strictly linear spoken and written codes. Last, but not least, it would be extremely beneficial for people who rely on nonverbal language systems for their communication, increasing the possibilities for their participation in school and the community.

There is no *a priori* reason why children with Down syndrome should be prevented from developing bilingual or even multilingual repertoires, even if it is unlikely that the levels of functioning eventually reached in the additional languages would be any different from that in the maternal tongue. Nor is it likely, as sometimes believed by some people – in our view naïvely – that bilingualism per se could alleviate some of the cognitive limitations inherent in Down syndrome. In other words, bilingualism may probably be encouraged in children with Down syndrome with some caution when it is part of the family or community situation, but it is neither a cognitive nor a language therapy.

Quite clearly, language intervention must be planned in an age-related manner. Early intervention (from birth, as we shall argue) is an absolute necessity (De Graaf, 1995). It carries the best hopes for lasting effects from prelinguistic skills on to later linguistic structures. It can meaningfully be carried out in close collaboration with the family of the infant and young child with Down syndrome. Continued intervention during schooling should be organized in association with the schools (see Beveridge, 1996). As language development occurs over time, particularly in individuals with Down syndrome, a series of linguistic structures to be improved can be proposed, in parallel with typical language acquisition, at each school level. Parents will often need to be advised on how to help their children effectively during the school years and how to make appropriate choices regarding curricular options (Rynders, 1994).

Another topic of importance relates to the peer relations of children with Down syndrome in mainstreamed groups. There one has children with Down syndrome and typically developing children at different developmental levels interacting with each other in classroom and play activities (see Guralnick, 1996; Guralnick, Connor, Hammoud, Gottman and Kinnish, 1996).

Intervention should also be recommended in late adolescence and early adult years, particularly with regard to the lexical, pragmatic and discursive aspects of language, which do not seem to exhibit critical period characteristics, as opposed to the phonological and morphosyntactic abilities, which do seem to be affected by critical periods (cf. Rondal and Edwards, 1997 for a full-scale discussion). It is highly advisable as a means of enhancing socio-cultural and work integration in individuals with Down syndrome (Rosenberg and Abbeduto, 1993). Lastly, language intervention with ageing persons with Down syndrome is not only possible but necessary. It should adapt current programmes with the elderly in the typical population. This could also provide a way to slow down language deterioration in the early stages of Alzheimer's disease in some with Down syndrome.

When designing language intervention programmes, individual differences have to be taken into account. Unfortunately, the study of these differences in intellectual disabilities (or in Down syndrome) is still little advanced. Current intervention work and programmes include nothing or only a little of this important dimension, despite lip service sometimes being paid to the issue. Exceptional cases of language development in individuals with Down syndrome and other intellectual disabilities have been specified in recent research (cf. Rondal, 1994, 1995, in press), suggesting that the variance may be quite large. Those working in the field of intellectual disabilities still have to incorporate fully the data on the range of individual differences and adapt their approaches accordingly.

It seems clear that interventions that take into account etiological characteristics have more chance of being effective. This claim was already formulated by Gibson (1981; see also Gibson, 1991 for additional specifications in the area of cognitive remediation). Dykens, Hodapp and Leckman (1994), Turk, Hagerman, Barnicoat and McEvoy (1994) and Dykens and Hodapp (2001) insist that patterns of development in individuals with intellectual disabilities may be, at least partly, syndrome specific. Professionals should try to tailor intervention to specific etiological groups. Regarding speech and language, Rondal (2001; see also Rondal and Comblain, 1999) has analysed the language profiles of six syndromes of genetic origin. This analysis shows considerable partial specificity across syndromes. Intervention programmes might work better when the child's etiology is among several important characteristics taken into account in designing remediation. The present work concentrates on Down syndrome and therefore feeds axiomatically on the specificity argument.

The effectiveness issue

Evaluating the effectiveness of an intervention, particularly a language intervention, is clearly a difficult task. The goal is to enhance the individual's learning of better linguistic structures and behaviours. Having acquired these, individuals ought to be able not only to produce or understand specific exemplars involving the learned structures but to exhibit generalized changes on given language aspects (Rusch and Karlan, 1983).

Studies that evaluate the effectiveness of language intervention are still too rare. At the end of their comprehensive review, Snyder-MacLean and MacLean (1987) suggested that language intervention can be only moderately effective in modifying the course of language development. Their somewhat negative position at the time (also relayed by Hauser-Cram, 1989, and Price, 1989) was largely motivated by considerations of the many difficult methodological, evaluative and even ethical problems (for example, who should be assigned to the experimental and/or the control groups?) in assessing remediation work – and by the fact that few of the published intervention studies at the time had provided systematic longitudinal data and/or data regarding the maintenance and the generalization of treatment effects to real-world communicative contexts. Warren and Kaiser (1988) argued that proper generalization and transfer of language intervention is rarely systematically explored and that it might even be considered that it is not usually achieved. According to these authors, proper generalization would be manifested as an increased rate of developmental progress after the intervention has reached a stringent criterion.

It is our opinion, indeed, that remediation programmes offered to children with moderate or severe intellectual disabilities have not met with sufficient success yet, particularly in fostering phonological, morphosyntactic, and discourse development. However, the areas of basic semantics and pragmatics, being more accessible and more easily accessed by language therapists and teachers, have begun to yield clearer gains and more stable ones, of course within the cognitive limits of individuals. Critical time periods for development in the conceptual aspects of language do not appear to exist, unlike in phonology and morphosyntax (Rondal and Edwards, 1997). This permits additional time and degrees of freedom for intervention. The areas of phonology and morphosyntax (so-called computational aspects of language) are technically more complex, demanding additional knowledge and professional skills from the therapist.

Yet, the general opinion of professionals in the field regarding at least the short- and middle-term efficiency of their practices with individuals with Down syndrome (particularly children) is generally positive, contrasting with the scepticism expressed in the judgements of the authors mentioned above. Beyond any undue naïveté it may be the case that more recent, methodologically sound, intervention strategies are yielding more positive outcomes. For example, programmes based on sound principles and involving parents or caretakers collaborating with professionals seem promising. Salmon, Rowan, and Mitchell (1998) have reported a positive impact of adult prompting in facilitating prelinguistic communication in toddlers with Down syndrome. Explicit prompting by interacting adults (as opposed to minimal prompting) had a marked effect in promoting higher overall rates of intentional communication in the children. Iacono, Chan and Waring (1998) had preschool children with Down syndrome and their mothers collaborating with a speech pathologist and special educator who acted as consultants within a collaborative consultation process aiming at defining and controlling the application of language-intervention strategies. Comparisons with a multiple baseline design demonstrated the efficiency of the intervention procedure for three out of the five children involved. Descriptive analyses of mothers' communicative behaviours indicated that, following treatment, they tended to direct more utterances to their children, model more, use more language-teaching strategies, ask fewer questions and produce fewer directives. That these improvements, although quite interesting, were not sufficient for progress was indicated by the fact that two out of the five target children failed to exhibit significant language improvement over time. Girolametto, Weitzman and Clements-Baartman (1998) have reported success in fostering expressive vocabulary development in young DS children, relying on parental involvement that promoted interaction and encouraged modelling and imitation of vocabulary (see also Girolametto, 2000).

Another promising aspect of recent intervention programmes is the increased attention devoted to prelinguistic communication as a way to prepare and positively affect the emergence of receptive and productive language in infants with Down syndrome (see also Chapter 2 in this book). Yoder and Warren (2001) have conducted a study on the treatment effects of prelinguistic communication interventions on language in toddlers with developmental delays. Only some of these children had Down syndrome. Others were premature with medical complications, had macrocephaly, neonatal meningitis, tuberous sclerosis, foetal alcohol syndrome, or no identifiable etiology or diagnosis other than serious developmental delay. Yoder and Warren (2001) report positive treatment effects on children's language development extending six and 12 months after the end of prelinguistic intervention (conducted four times a week for six months) and affecting important aspects of early language development such as comprehension of semantic relations, global measures of expressive and receptive language, and lexical density (the average rate of non-imitative vocabulary words used). The treatment outcomes, however, varied significantly as a function of pretreatment maternal responsiveness and educational level.

In a 25-chapter review, covering more than 35 years of research and practice in early intervention, Guralnick (1997) shows how far this field has come in solidifying the science of early intervention. This makes it clear that the efficiency of early intervention depends on complex and delicate interactions between programme objectives and features, and child and family characteristics. In the introduction to the book, Guralnick distinguishes 'first generation (i.e., till the late 1980s)' and 'second generation' early intervention research. The former is described as a period in which there was much concern about whether early intervention was indeed effective and worth doing and subsidizing. Second generation work extends beyond this question towards specifying empirically what characteristics of intervention are effective (or more effective) with particular pathological entities and particular groups of children and families, and understanding the mechanisms through which interventions operate. Of course, interventionists do not claim to cure children with intellectual disabilities, and therefore achieve therapy in the strict sense. Rather they aim to use the necessary knowledge and technological tools needed to give these children an advantage that may not have existed without intervention and to foster better development, particularly if intervention starts sufficiently early. It may indeed be considered that the work accomplished since the early 1970s provides the foundation for the next generation of intervention and prevention programmes and research, with the general objective of specifying effective remediation activities more precisely and increasing their long-term effects. In the same way, it is clear that future improvements in programme efficiency, the generalizability and durability of gains, will also depend on increased knowledge of the mechanisms and sequences characteristic of language development in the various etiologic entities causing intellectual disabilities.

References

Beveridge M (1996) School integration for Down's syndrome children: Policies, problems, and processes. In JA Rondal, J Perera, L Nadel, A Comblain (eds) Down's Syndrome: Psychological, Psychobiological and Socio-educational Perspectives. London: Whurr, pp. 207–18.

Cicchetti D, Beeghly M (1990) An organizational approach to the study of Down's syndrome: contributions to an integrated theory of development. In D Cicchetti, M Beeghly (eds), Children with Down's Syndrome: A Developmental Perspective. New York: Cambridge University Press, pp. 29–62.

Dykens E, Hodapp R (2001) Research in mental retardation: toward an etiologic approach. Journal of Child Psychology and Psychiatry 42: 49–71.

Dykens E, Hodapp R, Leckman J (1994) Behaviour and development in Fragile X syndrome. London: Sage.

Gibson D (1981) Down's Syndrome. The Psychology of Mongolism. Cambridge: Cambridge University Press.

Gibson D (1991) Down's syndrome and cognitive enhancement: Not like the others. In K Marfo (cd.) Early Intervention in Transition: Current Perspectives on Programs for Handicapped Children. New York: Praeger, pp. 61–90.

Girolametto L (2000) Participation parentale à un programme d'intervention précoce sur le développement du langage: Efficacité du programme parental de Hanen. Rééducation Orthophonique 203: 31–62.

Girolametto L, Weitzman E, Clements-Baartman J (1998) Vocabulary intervention for children with Down syndrome: parent training using focused stimulation. Infant-Toddler Intervention 8: 109–26.

Graaf E de (1995) Early intervention for children with Down's syndrome. In A. Vermeer and W. Davis (eds) Physical and Motor Development in Mental Retardation. Basel: Karger, pp. 120–43.

Guralnick, M (1996) Future directions in early intervention for children with Down's syndrome. In JA Rondal, J Perera, L Nadel, A Comblain (eds) Down's Syndrome: Psychological, Psychobiological and Socio-educational Perspectives. London: Whurr, pp. 147–62.

Guralnick M (ed.) (1997) The Effectiveness of Early Intervention. Baltimore Md: Brookes.

Guralnick M, Connor R, Hammoud M, Gottman J, Kinnish K (1996) The peer relations of preschool children with communication disorders. Child Development 67: 471–89.

Hauser-Cram P (1989) The efficiency of early intervention. Ab Initio 1: 1–2.

Iacono T, Chan J, Waring R (1998) Efficacy of a parent-implemented language intervention based on collaborative consultation. International Journal of Language and Communication Disorders 33: 281–303.

Price P (1989) Language intervention and mother–child interaction. In M Beveridge, G Conti-Ramsden, I Leudar (eds) Language and Communication in Mentally Handicapped People. London: Chapman & Hall, pp. 185–217.

Rondal JA (1994) Exceptional language development in mental retardation: natural experiments in language modularity. Current Psychology of Cognition 13: 427–67.

Rondal, JA (1995) Exceptional Language Development in Down Syndrome. Implications for the Cognition–language Relationship. New York: Cambridge University Press.

Rondal JA (in press) Atypical language development in mental retardation. Theoretical implications. In L Abbeduto (ed.) Language and Communication. International Review of Research in Mental Retardation. New York: Academic.

Rondal JA (2001) Language in mental retardation: individual and syndromic differences, and neurogenetic variation. Swiss Journal of Psychology 60: 161–78.

Rondal JA and Comblain A (1999) Current perspectives on developmental dysphasias. Journal of Neurolinguistics 12: 181–212.

Rondal JA, Edwards S (1997) Language in Mental Retardation. London: Whurr.

Rosenberg S, Abbeduto L (1993) Language and Communication in Mental Retardation. Development, Processes and Intervention. Hillsdale NJ: Erlbaum.

Rusch J, Karlan G (1983) Language training. In J Matson, J Mulick (eds) Handbook of Mental Retardation. New York: Pergamon, pp. 397–409.

Rynders J (1994). Supporting the education development and progress of individuals with Down's syndrome. Communication to the Third Ross Roundtable on Critical Issues in Family Medicine, Washington DC, July.

Salmon C, Rowan L, Mitchell P (1998). Facilitating prelinguistic communication: Impact of adult prompting. Infant-Toddler Intervention 8: 11–27.

Snyder-MacLean L, MacLean J (1987) Effectiveness of early intervention for children with language and communication disorders. In M Guralnick, F Bennett (eds) The Effectiveness of Early Intervention for At-risk and Handicapped Children. New York: Academic, pp. 213–74.

Turk J, Hagerman R, Barnicoat A, McEvoy J (1994) The fragile X syndrome. In N Bonras (ed.) Mental Health in Mental Retardation: Recent Advances and Practices. Cambridge: Cambridge University Press, pp. 135–53.

Warren S, Kaiser A (1988) Research in early language intervention. In S Docom, M Karnes (eds) Research in Early Childhood Special Education. Baltimore Md: Brookes, pp. 89–108.

Yoder P, Warren S (2001) Relative treatment effects of two prelinguistic communication interventions on language development in toddlers with developmental delays vary by maternal characteristics. Journal of Speech, Language, and Hearing Research 44: 224–37.

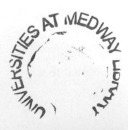

Chapter 2
Prelinguistic training

JEAN A RONDAL

Prelinguistic development covers most of the first 18 months of the life of the typically developing infant. The same development is extended in the child with Down syndrome and occupies most of the first two or three years. During this period, children learn the basic principles of human communication, first at the nonverbal level. They gradually go from a global mode of expression, involving the whole or most of the body, to more differentiated forms centring on vocal activity. The infant's vocal activity modifies itself considerably during prelinguistic development. It goes from crying and cooing to babbling, and later to the production of unconventional and then conventional words. The first year also witnesses a remarkable evolution in the mental activity of the infant. It evolves from physiological reflexes to a beginning of representation of the human and physical environment, major aspects of which have been described by authors such as Piaget (1936, 1937) and Spitz (1958). Spitz analysed the infant's evolution in the first year of life as concentrating on the construction of the affective figures. Other authors, such as Schaffer and Emerson (1964) and Yarrow (1972), have described the affective bonding process between mother and infant during the first year, and the appearance, at around 7 or 8 months in the infant, of the first reactions of fear in the presence of strangers. However, the infant's construction of the world does not concern only the affective figures. Piaget and others, particularly Bower, have analysed in great detail the infant's early representation of reality (see Piaget, 1937; Bower, 1967): for example, perceptual object permanence and the object permanence concept, as well as the evolution of what Piaget called sensorimotor intelligence (the intellectual regulations embodied in the baby's sensorimotor activities prior to symbolic development and language, corresponding to Vygotsky's notion of prelinguistic intelligence – Vygotsky, 1929, 1962).

During this period, infants organize their immediate physical world into more stable entities, which become targets for symbolic coding and vocal labelling. In the same way, they become sensitive to a number of typical relations between persons, objects, and events, which supply the basis for semantic relational development.

Towards the end of the first year or beginning of the second year, typically developing children understand a limited number of words and short multiword utterances in context. They are then close to trying to produce them. The symbolic link between significant and signified is within conceptual reach and will serve as a basis for further lexical development.

Sensorimotor development

Results of neurological examinations (see Cowie, 1970) show hypotonia and abnormalities in the early reflexes and automatisms of infants with Down syndrome. These include the palmar and plantar grasp reflexes, the Landau reaction (ventral suspension), the Moro response and automatic stepping. Retarded dissolution of early reflexes and reactions is also commonly observed in this syndrome. Motor development is delayed, mostly due to congenital hypotonia. As classically noted (for example by Paine, 1963) intellectual disabilities are often associated with generalized hypotonia. Problems in motor development in infants with moderate and severe intellectual disabilities may further delay early cognitive development to the extent that the latter is at least partly dependent upon moving around in a familiar physical setting, manipulating objects, and perceiving and acting on events and relationships between people and objects, objects and objects, people and people. Piaget (1936, 1937) claimed that the knowledge of young infants is framed in terms of the sensorimotor impressions familiar objects have on them and the motor adjustments the objects require. The child will not have verbal concepts until the second year of life.

Sound discrimination

By late foetal life, the hearing mechanism is normally well developed. It is believed that the foetus cannot hear sounds of normal intensity. However, it has the capacity to perceive sounds beyond 60 or 70 dB, particularly low-frequency sounds (also transmitted through bone vibration). Visual mechanisms are less well developed at birth than auditory ones. However, a full-term infant is able to follow visually a slowly moving object of medium size. He or she is sensitive to object contours and patterns within a few days of birth. Myelinization of the visual nervous fibres is not completed until several months after birth, and improvement in the ability to fixate accurately and to see details continues to take place until about 6 years of age.

As a result of prenatal and perinatal development, typically developing infants display early discrimination of their mothers' voice and speech, providing it is normally intonated. If the mother is requested to read sentences backwards, the infant no longer recognizes his or her mother's voice. Young typically developing infants are also able to discriminate their maternal language (in the double sense here of the language of the cultural community first heard and the mother's language) from any other language presented. Mehler, Lambertz, Jusczyk and Amiel-Tison (1987) presented random alternative sequences of 15-second speech samples from French and Russian to 4-day-old neonates. All could reliably differentiate maternal and foreign language as indicated by modifications induced in the rates of non-nutritive sucking (operated according to the paradigm of selective habituation). Such a discriminative performance is based on an analysis of the prosodic properties (and more specifically rhythmic characteristics) of the languages (cf. Nazzi, Bertoncini and Mehler's 1998 experiment with 5-day-old babies, and Dehaene-Lambertz and Houston's 1997 work with 2-month-old infants). However, the babies are able to discriminate two languages only if one of the two is already familiar. These observations mean that, from birth onwards, the human infant is sensitive to the prosodic characteristics of what will later be recognized as sentences belonging to the community language.

Most remarkable is the capacity of the young infant to perceive syllables (serially ordered binary sounds or triplets supplying the building blocks of speech, itself probably the most complex serially ordered behaviour in living forms). Syllables also play an important role in speech perception in many languages. They usually are discriminated better and with shorter response times by adults than single phonemes (for example, Savin and Bever, 1970). Young infants are capable of distinguishing syllables in alternating triplets of consonant – vowel – consonant (such as 'pat' versus 'bat'). Normal syllables shortened to 30-second stimuli can be reliably differentiated by neonates as opposed to 20 seconds for adults (Bertoncini, Bijeljac-Babic, Blumstein and Mehler, 1987). Processing syllables in maternal language therefore requires only minimal additional learning on the older infant's part.

In the early 1970s, the now classic research conducted by Eimas, Siqueland, Jusczyk and Vigorito (1971) revealed that young infants perceive language sounds in a categorial way, just like adults (language sounds are perceived in a discontinuous way with very narrow frontiers between each other – physically, of course, sounds constitute continuous series). Following on Eimas et al.'s work, researchers established that 1-month-old infants are potentially sensitive to the acoustic contrasts between many of the sounds existing in natural languages. For example, neonates are capable of discriminating between consonants on the basis of place of articulation (such as p, t, k) and mode of articulation (such as p, f) and oral vowels (such as a, i, u). A controversy subsists between universalists and developmentalists. The universalist position concludes from numerous studies that the infant's discriminative ability is excellent at birth and only some fine-tuning is necessary. The work of Eilers, Oller, Bull and Gavin (1984) and others suggests, however, that some particular contrasts may be correctly perceived only following some linguistic experience.

The neonates' overall discriminative ability for speech sounds gradually decreases over the first year of life, except for the phoneme sounds characteristic of their community language (or languages in multilingual situations). For example, Japanese babies are able to distinguish /r/ and /l/ sounds whereas older Japanese children and adults can no longer do this as these phonemes do not exist in the Japanese language. A number of longitudinal studies have been carried out in several languages (for example, Werker, Gilbert, Humphreys and Tees, 1981; Werker and Tees, 1984) showing that decreased discriminative ability for the phonemic contrasts that do not exist in the maternal language is established at around 10 to 12 months. The gradual loss of sensitivity to unheard phonetic contrasts seems to be cognitive and/or attentional but not neuro-sensory. Actually, as shown in a study by Best, McRoberts and Sithole (1988), there is no decrease in sensitivity in older infants for those sounds and contrasts that are not potential competitors for the phonemes of maternal language. Only those sounds and contrasts that share one or several dimensions with maternal phonemes are lost towards the end of the first year. The other sounds and contrasts with no equivalence or acoustic proximity in maternal language continue to be discriminated correctly in older children as well as in adults. It may be concluded that in the course of the first year there is receptive specialization aiming at establishing optimal discrimination of the phonemes of maternal language(s). This specialization is established on a statistical basis. The frequency of occurrence of the phonemes in a given language increases towards the centre part of the linguistic categories preferentially used in that language. Conversely, the less a given repertoire is practised, the lower is the frequency of occurrence of the sounds close to the basic phonemic categories. This explains why babies progressively ignore those sounds that have no distinctive value in their community language.

Babbling and infraphonological development

Indications corresponding to the evolution in sound discrimination have been reported regarding the evolution in typically developing babbling of infants over the first year. Oller and Lynch (1993) distinguish five major periods within babbling. They construct them as stages building upon each other towards adult speech sounds. Stage one (up to 2 months, approximately) witnesses reflex or quasi-reflex vocalizations with crying and other more-or-less vegetative sounds. Between approximately 2 and

4 months (stage two), babies produce cooing sounds tied to smiles and prevocalic phonetic structures. Oller (1990) observed a lengthening in duration of prevocalic and vocalic sounds between 3 and 4 months going from 700 to 1,400 milliseconds. In stage three (3 to 8 months), full pre-canonical (see below) babbling experience is going on. Researchers insist on the excellent ability of the typically developing infant to play with his or her voice, exploring its full range spectrum and contrastive power; producing a wide variety of sounds, for example quasi-vowels or immature vowel-like sounds, clicks, palatalized, rounded or pharyngeal consonants, affricates, sibilants, and so forth. A marked widening of the vocal spectrum is observed. Low-pitch (growls) as well as high-pitch (squeals) sounds may be produced beginning around the third month. The sounds produced by the infants also vary widely according to intensity level. Stage four (5 to 10 months) is characterized by the production of well-formed, or so-called canonical syllables, of the consonant (full) vowel (CV) type (for example, 'ba' or 'da'). Oller (1990) relates the concept of canonical syllable to that of minimal rhythmic unit of natural language, and its components, the nucleus, the margin(s), and the formant transition(s). Davis and MacNeilage (1994) interpret syllables in terms of a basic mouth opening–closing alternation, responsible for the typical vowel–consonant alternation of babbling. Oller and Eilers (1988) suggest that canonical syllabic babbling is first reduplicated (for example, 'mamama', 'papapapa', 'babababab' – which attests to a first clear auditory control over the vocal activity – and then variegated (consisting of consonants and vowels that differ). As observed by Steffens, Oller, Lynch and Urbano (1992), however, the production of pre-canonical syllables and quasi-vowels, although diminishing with time, persists into the second year of life. These data provide an indication that stage models such as Oller and Lynch's (1993) are idealizations, which may be useful, but that infants do not necessarily abandon previous vocal styles when moving ahead in development. Finally, stage five (9 to 18 months) witnesses the appearance of significant productions in the infant's babbling. It could be questioned whether this period is still babbling rather than pre-lexical or lexical as intended meaning begins to play a role in constraining vocal productions.

Before approximately 6 months, infants' babbling appears to be only minimally influenced by the community language. Sounds that do not belong to maternal language are produced. Between 6 and 12 months, an influence of the linguistic environment on phonetic characteristics of the infants' babbling is most likely. Konopczynski (1986), quoting from a unpublished work by Tuaycharoen, observes that as early as 6 months Thai babies' babbling differs at the prosodic level from the babbling of babies raised in non-tonal linguistic environments. Contradictory results have been reported by Oller and Eilers (1988), reporting no difference in the babbling of English and Spanish infants as well as other languages in the second half of the first year. However, a series of studies conducted by De Boysson-Bardies and associates (De Boysson-Bardies, Sagart and Durand, 1984; De Boysson-Bardies and Durand, 1991; Hallé, De Boysson-Bardies and Durand, 1992) clearly demonstrates the gradual influence of the community language on prosodic and segmental characteristics of infants' babbling in the second half of the first year.

These researchers have shown that phonetically naïve adults can reliably recognize prosodic features of their language (French, Algerian Arabic, or Cantonese) in 15-second babbling samples from 8- and 10-month infants. The existence of intonational differences between the reduplicative babbling of French- and English-learning infants (5 to 11 months) has been confirmed by Whalen, Levitt and Wang (1991). Such data corroborate the indication that typically developing infants begin to use prosodic features specific to their maternal language in the second half of the first year. De Boysson-Bardies and associates have demonstrated further that infants' babbling is differentiated according to segmental features circa 10 months of age. Vowel configurations from French, Algerian Arabic, and Cantonese infants, aged 10 months, were compared to speech sequences from adults of corresponding language communities for 'long-term spectrum'. Those spectra compute the spread of vocal energy for vocalic portions of speech signals lasting several minutes. The data reveal a good convergence between vowel characteristics of infant babbling and adult speech. This indication was confirmed in a direct analysis of the formant characteristics of the vowels produced in the babbling of 10-month infants exposed to French, English, Algerian Arabic, and Cantonese, respectively. It seems that the infants' vocalic space tends towards that of the adults towards the end of the first year. English-exposed infants and English-speaking adults have the highest formant two (oral)/formant one (pharyngeal) ratio observed, which corresponds to the prevalence in frequency of occurrence of diffuse vowels in English. Cantonese subjects produce the most compact vowels in average value. French and Algerian Arabic subjects are located in between the other two groups with formant one being lower in tonal value for the French subjects, which reflects the relatively high occurrence of closed rounded vowels in French (Hallé, Boysson-Bardies and Durand, 1992).

Babbling and speech perception in infants with Down syndrome

How do infants with Down syndrome develop prelinguistically in comparison to what is known of typically developing infants? Data are largely missing but some indications can be proposed. Dodd (1972) and Smith and Oller (1981) have suggested that the sounds of babbling are mostly similar in types and tokens in typically developing infants and infants with Down syndrome. Parameters such as number of vowel and consonant productions, number of non-speech noises, variety of consonants and vowels produced, length of vocalic and consonantal utterances, and general trends regarding the development of individual consonants and vowels, do not differentiate between the two groups of infants. However, syllabic patterning may be more problematic in infants with Down syndrome. In opposition to an earlier indication by Smith and Oller (1981), Lynch, Oller, Steffens, and Buder (1997) report that reduplicated babbling is delayed and less stable in infants with Down syndrome. The latter authors observe the onset of reduplicated babbling around 6 months at home and 9 months in laboratory studies in typically developing infants versus 8 and 10 months, respectively, in infants with Down syndrome. The discrepancies between the results of Lynch et al. (1997) and those of Smith and Oller (1981) may be due to differences in the frequency of contact between investigators and subjects. Lynch et al. (1997) sampled vocalizations more frequently.

Reduplicated babbling may be a distinct precursor to meaningful speech. In Lynch et al.'s (1997) study, the age of onset of reduplicated babbling estimated from parental report was significantly correlated with the score of the infants with Down syndrome at 27 months CA on the Early Social-Communication Scales (Mundy, Seibert and Hogan, 1984). These scales have predictive value with respect to subsequent development of verbal communication (Mundy, Sigman and Kasari, 1990). It seems to be the case that Down syndrome negatively influences expressive vocal development as early as the first year of life. Possible explanatory variables for the delays of infants with Down syndrome in the development of canonical syllables and reduplicated babbling are maturational delay, generalized hypotonia at birth and in the following months, and mild to moderate hearing loss in many of the babies. Over time, however (particularly in the first half of the second year of life), and in spite of marked individual differences, infants with Down syndrome increase their production of full vowels and canonical consonant–vowel syllables, implying better coordinated articulatory movements. They decrease their production of less mature quasi-vowels and pre-canonical syllables (Steffens, Oller, Lynch and Urbano, 1992).

Very few systematic data have been reported on speech perception in babies with Down syndrome and its evolution compared to typically developing babies. Eilers, Bull, Oller and Lewis (1985) have suggested that infants with Down syndrome may be limited in perceiving place of articulation distinctions in well-formed syllables. A problem with speed of auditory processing may be involved. Indeed when syllables were slowed down through synthesis of acoustic stimuli in Eilers et al.'s (1985) research, infants with Down syndrome showed improved performance. More research on these aspects of prelinguistic development in infants with Down syndrome is necessary. One needs to know the exact capacities of these babies regarding early recognition of mother's voice and maternal language, sensitivity to prosodic and rhythmic aspects of adult language, to pre-canonical and canonical syllables and related speech structures, the early differentiation of infra-phonemic contrasts, as well as the evolution of these abilities over time.

Interactive babbling

As early as 3 months, prelinguistic vocalizations may display particular characteristics labelled 'phrasing' (Lynch et al., 1997). Prelinguistic phrasing is defined as intermittent babbling, approximately three seconds long, characterized by the rhythm and structure that later underlie speech (for example, phrase-ending syllables last longer than other syllables, which can be interpreted as a signal prefigurating turn-taking organization). The DS babies (2 to 12 months of age) studied by Lynch et al. (1997) displayed the same rhythmic organization in prelinguistic phrases as typically developing infants. But they took longer to finish a prelinguistic phrase (an average of more than five seconds). This extended timeframe could explain why mothers and their babies with Down syndrome are often found to vocalize simultaneously (Jones, 1977; Buckhalt, Rutherford and Goldberg, 1978; Berger and Cunningham, 1983).

Infants with Down syndrome may be slower to develop prelinguistically. We need to specify better in which respects and why. Prelinguistic phrasing should be investigated carefully for it may provide an indication of the vocal exchange patterns that contribute to the developing bond between babies and people. This bond may be necessary for communication development.

Symbolic babbling

Typically developing children are known to produce jargon babbling (meaningless babbling sequences that sound like sentences because they reproduce the intonational structures of adult speech). The onset is 12 to 14 months (Petitto and Marentette, 1991). At about the same time, typically developing infants begin to produce particular sounds or sequences of sounds in order to refer to object entities or to suggest some course of action. Halliday (1975) has supplied examples of this stage from diary observations of his son Nigel. For example, Nigel had two early vocalized requests for joint action of the type expressed in adult language by 'let's'. These were the equivalent of the adult form 'let's go for a walk' and 'let's draw a picture'. The first was expressed by a sound of Nigel's 'invention', a very slow vibration of the vocal chords; the other a sound that at first was probably an imitation of the word 'draw', and later more often as 'bow-wow', meaning originally 'let's draw a dog', but then generalized to a sense of 'let's draw a picture'. Earlier in his vocal development, Nigel would typically comment on the presence of a plane flying overhead with a sound that was his imitation of the noise of the plane.

The point is that, at this stage, the infant is developing a temporarily stable relation between some sounds and meanings. These meanings are usually not something that can be easily glossed in terms of the adult language. They correspond to the infant's perception of an event or object, and the infant tries to mark these perceptions through the use of vocal sounds. Carter (1978) confirmed Halliday's observations in a longitudinal analysis of the communication acts of an infant between 12 and 24 months. She noted numerous examples of phonetically stable vocalizations containing elements of meaning. Golinkoff (1983) has stressed the interactive nature of such vocalizations. She demonstrated the role played by mothers' interpretation of the infant's proto-words and the true process of 'meaning negotiation' taking place between the partners in this type of interaction.

Few systematic observations are available on these developments in infants with Down syndrome. It is likely that object permanence and sensorimotor intellectual development are delayed in these infants in proportion to their cognitive handicap. Wishart (1993) has analysed individual developmental profiles drawn from a series of longitudinal studies of early cognitive development in children with Down syndrome. On the whole, age of initial acquisition of most object concept stages was found to lag only a few months behind control subjects. However, developmental instability was a recurrent theme. Cicchetti and Mans-Wagener (1987) also reported little delay in object permanence development in children with Down syndrome. Rast and Meltzoff (1995), on the contrary, signal a marked delay. Their typically developing infants reached high-level object permanence (invisible displacements) at about 8 to 12 months, which is consistent with the usual developmental indications (Piaget, 1936; Uzgiris and Hunt, 1975), whereas their children with Down syndrome ranged from approximately 20 to 43 months for the same acquisition. Rast and Meltzoff (1995) suggested that the studies reporting little delay in object permanence for children with Down syndrome actually provided training by testing the infants repeatedly. They find support for their hypothesis in the indication that positive outcomes in those studies were not maintained after termination of the regular testing schedule (Wishart, 1988).

Transition from babbling to speech production

It is now clear that infant vocalizations are continuous with later development of spoken language. The discontinuity hypothesis proposed by Jakobson (1941, 1968), Lenneberg, Rebelski, and Nichols (1965) and Lenneberg (1967), according to which prelinguistic vocalizations have no direct relationship with further language and only illustrate the maturation of the neurophysiological apparatus for speech, no longer finds persuasive defenders. It appears, on the contrary, that for typically developing infants at least, the phonetic characteristics of babbling persist into early word production and influence early word selection (Kent and Miolo, 1995). Prelinguistic development should certainly receive more attention from researchers for it could yield additional clues as to why the onset of conventional language is markedly delayed in children with Down syndrome (also Mundy and Sheinkopf, 1998). Despite the limited amount of information available, it is already possible to define a number of activities with the potential of improving prelinguistic development in infants with Down syndrome. They may be conveniently classified in seven sections:

- installing a reciprocal relation with the infant
- stimulating auditory and visual perception
- fostering nonverbal communication and gestural imitation
- stimulating babbling
- fostering practical knowledge of the immediate environment
- promoting symbolic games, and
- reducing buccal hypotonia and oro-facial dysfunctions.

I develop these points in the rest of the chapter (for more details, see my intervention guides: Rondal, 1986, 1987, 1998).

Installing a reciprocal relation

Probably the first structure to set in place, because it conditions the following ones, is the reciprocal relation between adult and infant. Reciprocity means that the partners in what becomes a genuine interaction act and react one with regard to the other and conversely. The initiating partner acts with the aim to elicit a reaction from the other person in the dyad. The second one reacts to the behaviour of the first one, and so forth. Behavioural reciprocity, including with the typically developing infant, at the beginning rests exclusively with the adult. It is gradually shared with the infant. This process is extended in time with the infant with Down syndrome and necessitates attention and help to speed it up.

Daily activities such as the alimentary, changing, clothing, and bathing routines are optimally suited for the installation and consolidation of reciprocal relations between caretakers and infant. They also contribute powerfully to supplying the infant with stable points of space and time reference in his or her world in construction. Often, infants with Down syndrome display lower frequencies of vocal and non-vocal requesting (Mundy and Sheinkopf, 1998). They need to be stimulated to exercise more communicative pressure on their social environment as a way to register themselves more actively in dyadic and gradually interactive episodes with more than one other person.

Stimulating auditory and visual perception

It is, of course, necessary to have the visual and the hearing acuity of the infant with Down syndrome carefully checked as soon as this is technically feasible within the first year of life. Precise information from the paediatric specialist will be useful to calibrate the intensity and the range of frequencies of the stimuli addressed to the baby with Down syndrome. Numerous activities can easily be programmed in order of increasing difficulty to be performed by the parents at home with the aim of increasing the child's sensitivity towards key physical dimensions of his or her immediately surrounding world. Visually, it is important to train the infant to gaze at particular persons, objects, and forms, analyse them perceptually, and follow their movements in space. Joint (child–adult) attention is of great importance too, for it is through the gaze of the caretaker that the young infant learns to explore substantial parts of the environment. Joint attention is not given at the start. It is largely a social construction, even in the typically developing child. In the infant with Down syndrome, it is usually delayed to an extent varying between individuals. Regarding auditory training, almost an infinity of sounds of various frequencies can be produced from familiar objects at varying intensities in order to stimulate the child and sensitize him or her to the acoustic properties of the immediate environment, the signaling value of a number of current life sounds and noises, and to develop the auditory discriminative ability.

It is always advisable to give parents extended information and, if possible practical demonstration, regarding the best ways to proceed prelinguistically with babies with Down syndrome.

Fostering nonverbal communication and gestural imitation

It is important for the parents and caretakers to identify and reinforce the expressive productions and communicative attempts of the infant with Down syndrome, for they supply the way towards babbling, then verbal, and later truly linguistic expression.

In the days following birth, caretakers should establish visual and body contact with the baby with Down syndrome, speak to him or her, of course not with the objective of communicating referentially but rather, and more importantly at that early stage, of empathic communication. One needs to touch the baby, caress him or her, make face-to-face contact, smile, and so forth. The child must realize as quickly as possible the social use he or she can make of the cries, body movements and gestures.

One can encourage children to learn to express themselves and to communicate using gestures through controlled activities of imitation, going from the imitation of simple facial expressions – for example, opening and closing mouth, protruding tongue, lips, closing the eyes, etc., to that of simple and then gradually more complex behaviours no longer directly connected to the face or the body.

Stimulating babbling

It is possible to distinguish several major stages in the evolution of babbling which also apply to the infant with Down syndrome (reflex vocalizations, prevocalic structures, precanoncial babbling, canonical babbling first reduplicated and then variegated). A more detailed scaling may be useful to follow the child's evolution more closely. I supply a list of steps characteristic of this evolution in Table 2.1. It is given as a mere example of what can be proposed to the parents, caretakers, and professionals with the hope of render them able to assist and promote babbling development in the infant with Down syndrome. Numerous checklists of the kind can be found in Rondal (1986, 1998). Such checklists have the advantage of serving, at the same time, as continuing assessment devices (allowing one at any time to precisely locate the level of evolution reached by the infant as to a particular aspect of it) and graduated intervention guides (aiming at promoting development). Step 2 in the list can and must be worked out or stimulated following attainment of step 1, and so on. Table 2.1 illustrates the babbling checklist.

Table 2.1. Babbling checklist (adapted from Rondal, 1986)

1. Child produces undifferentiated sounds, cries, and noises.
2. Child relies on one or several particular sounds, noises, or types of cries when claiming attention or requesting someone or something.
3. Child produces vowel-like or sounds but still difficult or impossible to identify clearly.
4. Child produces sounds (noises) close to consonants but still difficult or impossible to identify clearly.
5. Sounds close to middle vowels (e.g., [ae, a]) come to dominate in frequency.
6. Sounds close to front (e.g., [i, e]) and back vowels (e.g., [u, o]) are produced more frequently.
7. Palatal and velar consonants (e.g., [k, g]) dominant in frequency. They are produce in isolation or in the context of one vowel.
8. Labial consonants (e.g., [p, b, m]) increase in frequency, produced either in isolation within a vocalic context.
9. Babbling gradually increases its saturation in sounds characteristic of the community language.
10. The syllabic structuration of babbling becomes more obvious.
11. Reduplicated babbling appears (e.g., [mamama, papapa, tatata]).
12. Variegated babbling (vocal productions consisting of consonants and vowels that differ).
13. Prelinguistic phrasing (intermittent babbling a few seconds long with shortening of phrase-ending syllables).
14. Jargon babbling (i.e., meaningless sequences of syllables sounding like short sentences because they tend to mimic the basic intonational structures of adult speech acts.
15. Transition towards symbolic babbling (appearance of protowords).

Schemes of the above type can be easily explained to the parents and consulting professionals. Correctly understood and used they may constitute valuable tools for evaluating the infants' progress towards speech and guiding early training.

Fostering practical knowledge of the immediate environment

The infant with Down syndrome usually takes more developmental time to establish a strong eye contact with the mother (about three months on average). This is positive for mother–child bonding and for the exploration and discovery of the environment and actions surrounding the mother. It again takes longer than normal for the child with Down syndrome to reduce his or her high frequency of eye contact with the mother in order to start exploring visually the extramaternal environment, so to speak. Prelinguistic training should also aim at reducing as much as possible the delays in the infant's cognitive construction of the immediate world.

The first remedial task, after good levels of mother–child eye contact have been established and stabilized for a reasonable time, is to encourage extramaternal visual and then motor exploration of the familiar environment (following progression in motor development). Presenting the child with attractive, colourful and varied objects for sensory exploration will help in this development. Train the child to follow systematically the movements and displacements of the familiar adults in the room as well as, slightly later, the direction of the adult's gaze at certain moments. This second strategy, more demanding on the infant, will favour the establishment of joint attention between child and adult. Joint attention later will make it easier for the child to access coreference with the adult. Gazing together at the same object or event while the adult is labelling it or commenting on it, makes it possible for the child to guess correctly the meaning of the words uttered by the adult in practical situations and 'here and now' communication.

Another aspect of prelinguistic training concerns the gradual building of a repertoire of cognitive relations between persons and objects, persons and persons, objects and objects, events, and so forth, which will then serve as a basis for the development of the major semantic relations necessary for combinatorial language development – notions such as presence, disappearance, recurrence, qualitative and quantitative attribution, location in space, benefit, instrumentation, agent–action, action–object, agent–action, location, and agent–action–object. Numerous play activities are readily imaginable to favour development of these notions with the young child with Down syndrome.

Cognitive object permanence – the recognition that a given object continues to exist physically (within a matrix of spatial coordinates and relations) even when absent according to the senses, has long been considered a key step in early development. It is particularly important as a component of the referential process in first vocabulary development. The child has to realize that the words of the community language refer to entities persons, objects, events, that are stable in time and in space (at least to some reasonable extent), which makes it worth, functionally speaking, labelling them.

Table 2.2 supplies a checklist that can be used to promote object permanence development in the DS infant.

Promoting symbolic games

A linguistic sign or symbol associates a meaning (concept) with a form (coordinated sequence of phonemes) in a referential relationship with objects, persons or events. The association between form and meaning can be arbitrary or motivated. Arbitrary signs constitute the vast majority of the lexical repertoires of our languages. Arbitrariness means that there is no necessary relation between form and meaning (signifying and signified). In motivated signs (for example, onomatopeia and a few words), the relationship between meaning and form cannot be easily changed. Sign arbitrariness has the consequence that almost all form–meaning associations in a given language must be learned individually. They cannot be deduced in any easy way.

Before starting lexical development, the young child has to realize an important dimension of the word game – the symbolic mechanism that underlies all lexical acquisition. The key aspect of symbolism resides in a substitution principle: the possibility of replacing any class of entities by a 'portable' substitute ('quid pro quo', in the phrasing of the ancient philosophers – 'something to represent something else'). This principle, although simple, has proved extraordinary useful and powerful in the story of civilization. It is, of course, basic to any linguistic expression. The child has to rediscover it in the course of his or her early development. The symbolic principle is intrinsically cognitive. As such, delays can be expected and are currently observed in the development of the child with intellectual disabilities.

This developmental aspect, therefore, can be defined as a target for early intervention with the infant with Down syndrome. An interesting observation in typical development is that proto-words and the first beginning of lexical development are usually contemporaneous with symbolic play or 'let's pretend' play and activities. The child may spontaneously, for instance, place his or her head on a pillow or any flat surface and pretend to be sleeping, or do the same with a baby-toy or an animal-toy. Or he or she might close and open alternately the hand to imitate (symbolize) the closing–opening of a door, a window, or a matchbox (as observed long ago by Piaget with his own young children). These are motivated signs or symbols. The move toward arbitrary signs will take place in the very process of lexical development.

Table 2.2. Object permanence checklist (adapted from Rondal, 1986)

1.	*Object fixation*
1.1.	Child gazes at a non-moving object of average size for 3 seconds.
1.2.	Child gazes at a non-moving object of small size for 3 seconds.
1.3.	Child gazes at a non-moving object of average size for more than 3 seconds.
1.4.	Child gazes at a non-moving object of small size for more than 3 seconds.
1.5.	Child gazes at an object moving horizontally from the centre of the visual field to the periphery.
1.6.	Child gazes at an object moving horizontally from periphery to the centre of the visual field.
1.7.	Child gazes at a first object but switches his or her gaze towards a second object entering the visual field.
1.8.	Child switches his or her gaze alternately from one object to a second one present in the visual field.
2.	*Visual pursuit*
2.1.	Child follows visually an object moving horizontally.
2.2.	Child follows visually an object moving vertically.
2.3.	Child follows visually an object moving irregularly.
2.4.	Child follows visually an object disappearing behind a screen. Turns head and adapts body position in such a way as to ensure continued perception of the object as much as possible.
2.5.	Child follows visually an object passing behind him or her. Turns head towards the side where the object reappears.
3.	*Object search*
3.1.	Child explores visually (and possibly otherwise) the place where the object has disappeared (e.g., behind screen).
3.2.	Child gazes at and moves towards the place where the object can be expected to reappear.
3.3.	Child can retrieve immediately an object partially hidden behind a screen.
3.4.	Child can retrieve immediately an object completely hidden but put there in view of the child.
3.5.	Child plays hide and seek with familiar objects or persons.
3.6.	Child sees the adult hiding an object behind one of two screens. Can retrieve the object in one trial.
3.7.	Child sees the adult hiding an object behind one of three screens. Can retrieve the object in one trial.
3.8.	Adult shows one object to the child then hides it behind one of two screens. Child is able to retrieve the object in two trials maximum.
3.9.	Same as 3.8 but with three screens. Child is able to retrieve the object in three trials maximum.
3.10.	Three screens. The adult shows one object to the child, then hides it in his (her) hand, passes behind the three screen successively without releasing the object (child cannot see the adult's movement behind the screens). Child is able to search behind the screens for the object and then to retrieve it from the hand of the adult.

There are good reasons to believe that one needs to stimulate symbolic playing and symbolic activities in the child with Down syndrome as a

plausible way to promote proto-words and then conventional lexical development. A developmental review by Beeghly (1998) highlights the finding that the ontogeny of symbolic play is strongly associated with a basic social-communication system. This is quite logically so but, in children with Down syndrome particularly, it remains that the elaboration of symbolic activities has to be particularly encouraged if one wants to have a chance to reduce the important delays usually observed in that respect.

Reducing buccal hypotonia and oro-facial dysfunctions

Motor development in Down syndrome is closely associated with the degree of generalized hypotonia in these children (Poo and Gassio, 2000). The motor component of speech, therefore, can be expected to be more problematic in this syndrome. Several techniques have been designed in order to reduce buccal (particularly lingual) hypotonia in infants with Down syndrome. One of the best known techniques in this respect is that of Castillo-Morales, Avalle and Schmid (1984). It relies on the case of a palatal plate equipped with mechanical stimulators. The plate is placed in the mouth of the infant under the tongue. The anterior part of the plate stimulates the tongue and the articulatory muscles and activates the tonus of the lips. The posterior part of the plate stimulates the muscular tonus of the posterior part of the tongue and in so doing favours its positioning more backward in the mouth. The inferior lip, free of the tongue pressure upon it, can move more easily towards the upper lip, allowing oral occlusion. The average length of treatment according to Castillo-Morales et al. (1984) is 18 months. Placement of the plate is advised from 2 or 3 months of age. It can be used for periods of five to ten minutes, two or three times a day during the waking hours of the infant with Down syndrome. The plate has to be replaced every three or four months and modified to fit the growth of the mouth and the teeth in the infant.

Despite its relative efficiency (from 50% to 80% of reported success with groups of infants with Down syndrome, Williams syndrome, or cerebral palsy – Martin et al., 1996) the major problem with the Castillo-Morales plate is that its placement, removal, and keeping it in the mouth, are not that easy for the child and his or her caretakers. It is also not to be left in the child's mouth during sleep for reason of safety. De Andrade, Tavares, Rebelo, Palha and Tavares (1998) have designed a modified plate build like the Castillo-Morales but with the clever adjunction of a pacifier mechanically tied to the palatal plate. This new device has the advantage, among other things, of permitting a significantly longer positioning in the baby's mouth with the consequence of insuring a higher efficiency of the technique regarding the improvement of buccal hypotonia. De Andrade et al. (1998) insist, however, that their technique should optimally be combined with programmes of body and orofacial stimulation aimed at reducing lingual hypotonia and protrusion, labial hypotonia, and permanent mouth opening, whenever observed.

In some (fortunately) rare cases of important macroglossia, the above treatments may not suffice to insure the establishment of a proper speech apparatus in the child with Down syndrome. A surgical treatment has been available for a quarter of a century (e.g. Lemperle, 1985). It consists in removing a part of the lingual mass, taking care not to damage the taste buds on the surface and the anterior portion of the tongue. Such a treatment is advisable in only a minority of cases presenting an important macroglossia combined with a relatively small buccal cavity and lingual protrusion. Correctly performed it may improve the lingual-buccal apparatus and, in so doing, may facilitate pre-speech and speech training.

References

Beeghly M (1998) Emergence of symbolic play: perspectives from typical and atypical development. In J Burack, R Hodapp, E Zigler (eds) Handbook of Mental Retardation and Development. New York: Cambridge University Press, pp. 240–89.

Berger J, Cunningham C (1983) The development of early vocal behaviours and interactions in Down syndrome and non-handicaped infant–mother. Developmental Psychology 19: 322–31.

Bertoncini J, Bijeljac-Babic R, Blumstein S, Mehler J (1987) Discrimination of very short CVs in neonates. Journal of the Acoustical Society of America 82: 1–37.

Best C, McRoberts G, Sithole N (1988) Examination of perceptual reorganization for nonnative speech contrasts: Zulu click discrimination by English-speaking adults and infants. Journal of Experimental Psychology: Human perception and performance 14: 345–60.

Bower T (1967) The development of object-permanence: some studies of existence constancy. Perception and Psychophysics 2: 411–18.

Buckhalt J, Rutherford R, Goldberg I (1978) Verbal and non-verbal interaction of mothers with their Down's syndrome and non-retarded infants. American Journal of Mental Deficiency 82: 337–43.

Carter A (1978) From sensori-motor vocalizations to words: a case study of the evolution of attention-directing communication in the second year. In A Lock (ed.) Gesture and Symbol: The Emergence of Language. New York: Academic, pp. 126–48.

Castillo-Morales R, Avalle C, Schmid R (1984) Possibilità di trattamento della patologia orofaciale nella sindrome di Down con la placa di regolazione motoria. Pediatria Preventiva e Sociale 34: 1–4.

Cicchetti D, Mans-Wagener L (1987) Sequences, stages, and structures in the organization of cognitive development in infants with Down syndrome. In I Uzgiris, J Hunt (eds) Infant performance and experience: new findings with the ordinal scales. Urbana Ill: University of Illinois Press, pp. 281–310.

Cowie V (1970) A Study of the Early Development of Mongols. London: Pergamon.

Davis B, MacNeilage P (1994) Organization of babbling: a case study. Language and Speech 37: 341–55.

De Andrade D, Tavares P, Rebelo P, Palha M, Tavares M (1998) Placa modificada para tratamento de hipotonia oro-muscular em crianças com i dade compreendida entre os 2 meses e os 2 anos. Ortodontia 3(2): 111–17.

De Boysson-Bardies B, Durand C (1991) Tendances générales et influence de la langue maternelle dans le babillage et les premiers mots. L'Année Psychologique 91: 139–57.

De Boysson-Bardies B, Sagart L, Durand C (1984) Discernible differences in the babbling of infants according to target language. Journal of Child Language 11: 1–15.

Dehaene-Lambertz G, Houston D (1997) Faster orientation latencies toward native language in two-month-old infants. Language and Speech 41: 21–43.

Dodd B (1972) Comparison of babbling patterns in normal and Down's syndrome infants. Journal of Mental Deficiency 16: 35–40.

Eilers R, Bull D, Oller D, Lewis D (1985) The discrimination of rapid spectral speech cues by Down syndrome and normally developing infants. In S Harel, N Anastasiow (eds) The At-risk Infant. Psycho/Social/Medical Aspects. Baltimore: Brookes, pp. 115–32.

Eilers R, Oller D, Bull D, Gavin W (1984) Linguistic experience and infant perception. Journal of Child Language 11: 467–75.

Eimas P, Siqueland E, Jusczyk P, Vigorito J (1971) Speech perception in infants. Science 171: 303–6.

Golinkoff R (1983) The preverbal negotiation of failed messages: insights into the transition period. In R Golinkoff (ed.) The transition from prelinguistic to linguistic communication. Hillsdale NJ: Erlbaum, pp. 42–63.

Hallé K, De Boysson-Bardies B, Durand C (1992) Babillages et premiers mots. Glossa 29: 4–15.

Halliday M (1975) Learning how to Mean. Explorations in the Development of Language. London: Arnold.

Jakobson R (1941, 1968) Kindersprache, aphasie, und allgemeine lautgesetze. Uppsala: Almqvist & Wiksell (translated into English under the title Child Language, Aphasia, and Phonological Universals. The Hague: Mouton).

Jones O (1977) Mother–child communication with prelinguistic Down's syndrome and normal infants. In H Schaffer (ed.) Studies in Mother–infant Interaction. New York: Academic, pp. 126–49.

Kent R, Miolo G (1995) Phonetic abilities in the first year of life. In P Fletcher, B MacWhinney (eds) The Handbook of Child Language. Oxford: Blackwell, pp. 303–34.

Konopczynski, G. (1986). Du prélangage au langage: Acquisition de la structure prosodique. Unpublished doctoral dissertation, University of Strasbourg, France.

Lemperle G (1985) Plastic surgery. In D Lane, B Stratford (eds) Current Approaches to Down's Syndrome. London: Cassell, pp. 131–45.

Lenneberg E (1967) Biological Foundations of Language. New York: Wiley.

Lenneberg E, Rebelski F, Nichols I (1965) The vocalizations of infants born to deaf and to hearing parents. Human Development 8: 23–37.

Lynch M, Oller D, Steffens M, Buder E (1997) Phrasing in prelinguistic vocalizations. Developmental Psychology 33: 814–24.

Martin M, Vasquez E, Diz P, Figueiral H, Vasconcelos L, Figueiredo J, De Andrade D (1996) Terapia de estimulaçao orofacial: Principios e consideraçoes. Revista de Saude Oral 12: 151–4.

Mehler J, Lambertz G, Jusczyk P, Amiel-Tison C (1987) Discrimination de la langue maternelle par le nouveau-né. Comptes-rendus de l'Académie des Sciences de Paris 303: 637–40.

Mundy P, Seibert J, Hogan A (1984) Relationship between sensorimotor and early communication abilities in developmentally delayed children. Merrill-Palmer Quarterly 30: 33–48.

Mundy P, Sheinkopf S (1998) Early communication skill acquisition and developmental disorders. In J Burack, R Hodapp, Zigler (eds) Handbook of Mental Retardation and Development. New York: Cambridge University Press, pp. 183–207.

Mundy P, Sigman M, Kasari C (1990) A longitudinal study of joint attention and language development in autistic children. Journal of Autism and Developmental Disorders 20: 115–28.

Nazzi T, Bertoncini J, Mehler J (1998) Language discrimination by newborns: toward an understanding of the role of rhythm. Journal of Experimental Psychology: Human Perception and Performance 24: 756–66.

Oller K (1990) The emergence of sounds in speech in infancy. In J Yeni-Komshian, J Kavanagh, C Ferguson (eds) Child Phonology. New York: Springer, vol. 1, pp. 93–112.

Oller K, Eilers R (1988) The role of audition in infant babbling. Child Development 59: 441–9.

Oller K, Lynch M (1993) Infant vocalizations and innovations in infraphonology: toward a broader theory of development and disorders. In C Ferguson, L Menn, C Stoel-Gammon (eds) Phonological Development. Parkton Md: York Press, pp. 509–36.

Paine R (1963) The future of the 'floppy infant': a follow-up study of 133 patients. Developmental Medicine and Child Neurology 5: 115–24.

Petitto A, Marentette P (1991) Babbling in the manual mode: evidence for the ontogeny of language. Science 251: 1493–6.

Piaget J (1936) La Naissance de l'Intelligence chez l'Enfant. Neuchâtel: Delachaux et Niestlé.

Piaget J (1937) La construction du réel chez l'enfant. Neuchâtel: Delachaux et Niestlé.

Poo P, Gassio R (2000) Desarollo motor en ninos con sindrome de Down. Revista Medica Interacional sobre el Sindrome de Down 4(3): 34–40.

Rast M, Meltzoff A (1995) Memory and representation in young children with Down syndrome: exploring deferred imitation and object permanence. Development and Psychopathology 7: 393–407.

Rondal JA (1986) Le développement du langage chez l'enfant trisomique 21. Manuel pratique d'intervention. Bruxelles: Mardaga.

Rondal JA (1987) Faite parler l'enfant retardé mental. Un programme d'intervention psycholinguistique. Bruxelles: Cabor.

Rondal JA (1998) Educar y hacer a hablar al niño Down. Una guia al servicio de padres y profesores. Mexico DF: Trillas.

Savin H, Bever T (1970) The nonperceptual reality of the phoneme. Journal of Verbal Learning and Verbal Behavior, 9: 295–302.

Schaffer H, Emerson P (1964) The Development of Social Attachment in Infancy. Philadelphia: Monographs of the Society for Research in Child Development.

Smith B, Oller K (1981) A comparative study of pre-meaningfull vocalizations produced by normally developing and Down's syndrome infants. Journal of Speech and Hearing Disorders 46: 46–51.

Spitz R (1958) La Première Année de Vie de l'Enfant. Paris: Presses Universitaires de France.

Steffens M, Oller D, Lynch M, Urbano R (1992) Vocal development in infants with Down syndrome and infants who are developing normally. American Journal on Mental Retardation 97: 235–46.

Uzgiris I, Hunt J (1975) Assessment in infancy: ordinal scales of psychological development. Urbana Ill: University of Illinois Press.

Vygotsky L (1962) Thought and Language. Cambridge, Mass: MIT Press (first publication in Russian, 1929).

Werker J, Gilbert J, Humphreys G, Tees R (1981) Developmental aspects of cross-language speech perception. Child Development 52: 349–55.

Werker J, Tees R (1984) Cross-language speech perception: evidence for perceptual reorganization during the first year of life. Infant Behavior and Development 7: 49–63.

Whalen D, Levitt A, Wang Q (1991) Intonational differences between the reduplicative babbling of French- and English-learning, infants. Journal of Child Language 18: 501–16.

Wishart J (1988) Early learning in infants and young children with Down syndrome. In L Nadel (ed.) The Psychobiology of Down Syndrome. Cambridge Mass: MIT Press, pp. 7–50.

Wishart J (1993) The development of learning difficulties in children with Down's syndrome. Journal of Intellectual Disability Research 37: 389–403.

Yarrow L (1972) Attachment and dependency. In J Gewirtz (ed.) Attachment and Dependency. New York: Winston, pp. 81–95.

Chapter 3
Phonological working memory difficulty and related interventions

FRANCES A CONNERS

What difficulties do individuals with Down syndrome experience in memory? The list may seem long. People with Down syndrome typically fall in the low range of intellectual functioning, which implies that they have difficulties with many aspects of cognitive processing, including memory. However, the cognitive profile associated with Down syndrome suggests that phonological working memory is a specific relative weakness in this population (Chapman and Hesketh, 2000; Wang, 1996). This means that phonological working memory is weak relative to general intellectual functioning, and that this relative weakness is characteristic of Down syndrome relative to other etiologies associated with low intellectual functioning (see Jarrold, Baddeley and Phillips, 1999).

Phonological working memory serves to store speech-based information temporarily and process it along with information that has been retrieved from long-term memory. It is critical in any process that involves speech-coded information, particularly when the task involves a heavy information load and/or is cognitively effortful. Effortful learning of factual information and skills via verbal explanation or instruction relies heavily on phonological working memory. Clearly, a weakness in this important memory component can affect the development of language and reading skills as well as general knowledge base. Thus, intervention research related to phonological working memory is of critical importance.

In the first part of this chapter, I present evidence for a specific relative weakness in phonological working memory in Down syndrome. In the second part, I discuss interventions aimed at improving phonological working memory in individuals with Down syndrome. The few intervention studies that have been published show improvements, but the improvements are limited in scope and in durability. Thus, in the final part of the chapter, I suggest that an analysis of the locus of the phono-logical working memory deficit would help in the design of the next phase of interventions. I suggest directions for future research and inter-ventions.

Phonological working memory: a specific relative weakness

The evidence for a specific relative weakness in phonological working memory comes from two types of studies. In the first type, researchers used psychometric tests to identify areas of cognitive strengths and weak-nesses in people with Down syndrome. These studies included a wide variety of subtests and scales and produced highly consistent results showing a relative weakness in phonological working memory (often referred to in early studies as auditory short-term memory). In the second type of study, researchers used targeted experimental measures to further document the relative weakness in phonological working memory and to explore the nature of this weakness. In the present section I discuss evi-dence from these two types of studies. If phonological working memory is a specific relative weakness in Down syndrome, it would be

- weaker than other cognitive abilities in individuals with Down syn-drome
- weaker in individuals with Down syndrome than in typically develop-ing children who are of the same mental age level, and
- weaker in individuals with Down syndrome than in other individuals who have an intellectual disability of the same severity but do not have Down syndrome.

Also when individuals with Down syndrome are compared with other intellectual disability and typically developing groups, there should be abilities other than phonological working memory on which the groups are equivalent.

Studies using psychometric tests reported scores on the Illinois Test of Psycholinguistic Abilities (ITPA), The Kaufman Assessment Battery for Children (KABC), the McCarthy Scales of Children's Abilities (MSCA), and the Stanford-Binet 4 (SB4). On the ITPA, the Auditory Sequential Memory subtest best reflects phonological working memory. Individuals with Down syndrome scored low on Auditory Sequential Memory and Grammatical Closure relative to their own general level of performance, and scored high on Visual Closure (Bilovsky and Share, 1965; see also Marcell and Armstrong, 1982). They scored lower than typically develop-ing and other intellectual disability groups on Auditory Sequential Memory and Grammatical Closure as well as on Auditory Reception and Auditory Association, which involve phonological working memory (Burr and Rohr, 1978; Rohr and Burr, 1978; see also Prior, 1977; see Mackenzie and Hulme, 1987 for mixed results). On the KABC and similar tests of simultaneous and sequential processing, individuals with Down syndrome scored lower than typically developing comparison groups (Pueschel, Gallagher, Zartler and Pezzullo, 1987) and intellectual disability groups (Snart, O'Grady and Das, 1982) on the sequential scale. The sequential scale subtests involving phonological working memory were largely responsible for the differences. These were Number Recall and Word Order in the Pueschel et al. (1987) study, and Digit Span and Auditory Serial Recall in the Snart et al. (1982) study.

On the MSCA, children with Down syndrome scored lower than age- and IQ-matched children with Williams syndrome on the verbal and memory domains, better on the perceptual-performance domain, and the same on the quantitative domain (Klein and Mervis, 1999). In the memory domain, it was the phonological working memory subtests – verbal memory and numerical memory – that distinguished the groups; there was no difference in pictorial memory or tapping sequence. Finally, on the SB4, children with Down syndrome scored lower than other children with intellectual disabilities on the short-term memory scale (Bower and Hayes, 1994). Again, the phonological working memory subtests – memory for sentences and memory for digits – were responsible for the difference. There was no group difference on bead memory or memory for objects.

Studies using targeted experimental measures provided the same conclusion as the studies using psychometric tests. In several of the targeted studies, digit span or word span tasks were presented either aurally or visually to groups of individuals with and without Down syndrome. Individuals with Down syndrome performed more poorly on the aurally presented task but equivalently on the visually presented task compared with typically developing groups (Hulme and Mackenzie, 1992; McDade and Adler, 1980; Marcell and Weeks, 1988) and intellectual disability groups (Marcell and Weeks, 1988; Marcell Ridgeway, Sewell and Whelan, 1995; Marcell, Harvey and Cothran, 1988; see also Rondal, Lambert and Sohier, 1981). Moreover, when individuals with Down syndrome were matched with typically developing children on visual memory, the group with Down syndrome performed worse on auditory digit span and story recall (Kay-Raining Bird and Chapman, 1994). It should be noted that two studies in this group failed to find a difference between their Down syndrome group and their intellectual disability group on auditory working memory tasks (Hulme and Mackenzie, 1992; Varnhagan, Das and Varnhagan, 1987).

The targeted studies also showed that individuals with Down syndrome do not display the typical modality effect in which memory is better when verbal materials are presented aurally than when presented visually. Marcell and Weeks (1988) demonstrated this pattern comparing adolescents with Down syndrome with typically developing and intellectual disability comparison groups. Only the adolescents with Down syndrome showed no auditory modality advantage. Several other studies also showed no modality effect in individuals with Down syndrome (for example, Marcell and Armstrong, 1982; Marcell et al., 1988; McDade and Adler, 1980; Varnhagan et al., 1987) or even a visual modality advantage (Broadley, MacDonald and Buckley, 1995; Laws, MacDonald, Buckley and Broadley, 1995). Laws, et al. (1995) reported no modality effect for children with Down syndrome early on in their three-year study and a visual modality advantage at the end.

More recently, researchers have framed the phonological working memory deficit in terms of Baddeley's multicomponent model of working memory (Baddeley, 1986; Baddeley and Hitch, 1974; 1994). This model includes central executive, visuo-spatial, and phonological components, and allows us to look within the phonological component for specific problems. But does the evidence of performance difficulties with auditory versus visual presentation in working memory tasks fit into this framework? In most of the studies just discussed, verbal material (digits or words) was used in both the visual and auditory presentations. According to Baddeley's model, adults without intellectual disability would use the phonological loop to process information in both modalities because the information is naturally coded in a speech-based code. Much of the literature supporting the notion of the phonological loop shows the similarities of results for verbal materials whether presented aurally or visually (see Baddeley, 1986). However, the developmental literature suggests that it may take until the age of 7 to 10 years before children recode visual material into phonological codes (Hitch, Halliday, Schaafstal and Schraagen, 1988; Hitch, Woodin and Baker, 1989). Presumably, it would be at about this age when they begin to use the phonological loop to process verbal material that was presented visually. For individuals with Down syndrome or intellectual disability, it may take until a *mental* age of 7 to 10 years before recoding occurs systematically. In the studies just reviewed, the mental age of participants was nearly always below 7 years. Thus, the studies that compared auditory and visual presentations in young people with Down syndrome may indeed have compared phonological working memory with visuo-spatial working memory.

A set of recent studies guided by Baddeley's model more clearly measured phonological and visuo-spatial working memory. They compared performance on a digit span or word span task with performance on the Corsi span task. Each task begins with a short list that the participant tries to recall in the correct order. If performance is good, the task continues with a longer list, until the participant begins to make errors. The digit span and word span tasks involve verbal stimuli presented aurally. The Corsi span task consists of a series of spatial locations of blocks or squares presented visually. Most studies comparing individuals with Down syndrome with typically developing and intellectual disability comparison groups showed that those with Down syndrome had shorter digit/word spans and equivalent Corsi spans (Jarrold and Baddeley, 1997; Jarrold, Baddeley and Hewes, 1999, 2000; Marcell and Cohen, 1992; but see Vicari, Carlesimo and Caltagirone, 1995). Consistent with this pattern, individuals with Down syndrome had shorter digit spans but longer Corsi spans than individuals with Williams syndrome (Jarrold et al., 1999; Wang and Bellugi, 1994). Individuals with Down syndrome also had longer Corsi spans than individuals with fragile X, though the results for digit span are mixed (Crowe and Hay, 1990; Schapiro et al., 1995).

Thus, with a few exceptions, the evidence strongly points to a specific weakness in phonological working memory related to Down syndrome. Indeed, several alternative explanations of the 'specific weakness' have been investigated and ruled out. For example, poor hearing in individuals with Down syndrome does not account for poor performance on digit/word span tasks. Performance was poor compared to typically developing and intellectual disability comparison groups even in studies that screened out participants with hearing problems (Kay-Raining Bird and Chapman, 1994; Marcel and Armstrong, 1982; Marcell and Weeks, 1988; McDade and Adler, 1980), and even in studies that demonstrated that speech hearing acuity did not correlate with digit/word span (Jarrold et al., 2000; Marcel and Cohen, 1992; r = 0.05 and 0.06, respectively). Poor speech articulation in individuals with Down syndrome does not account for poor performance on digit/word span tasks. Performance was poor compared to typically developing and intellectual disability comparison groups even when manual rather than verbal responses were required (Jarrold et al., 2000; Marcell and Weeks, 1988). Distractibility of individuals with Down syndrome cannot account for their poor performance on digit/word span tasks. Eliminating distracting stimuli by using earphones or goggles did not change the results (Marcell et al., 1988). Finally, a general sequential processing difficulty cannot account for the poor performance on digit/word span tasks. Individuals with Down syndrome did not experience relative difficulties across a variety of sequential processing measures (Kay-Raining Bird and Chapman, 1994; Marcell and Armstrong, 1982; Pueschel et al., 1987; Snart et al., 1982; Varnhagan et al., 1987).

It is well known that phonological working memory is related to language development in the general population (see Gathercole and Baddeley, 1993). Studies on Down syndrome have also established this relationship, showing that measures of phonological working memory correlate with language measures such as grammatical comprehension and expressive language ability, and reading (Laws, 1998; Marcell et al., 1995; Rondal et al., 1981). Thus, there is a clear need to investigate interventions for individuals with Down syndrome targeted at improving phonological working memory.

Interventions targeting phonological working memory

In the early 1970s, researchers identified short-term memory deficits in individuals with intellectual disability of unknown or mixed etiology (for example Ellis, 1970). When these individuals were allowed to study, at their own pace, items that were to be recalled, researchers found that they did not show the same pattern of study times across serial position as shown by individuals without intellectual disability (for example, Belmont and Butterfield, 1969). Further, when the individuals with intellectual disability were trained to study the items the way the others did, they improved their recall (Belmont and Butterfield, 1969; Brown, Campione, Bray and Wilcox, 1973; Conroy, 1978; Hulme and Mackenzie, 1992; Kellas, Ashcraft and Johnson, 1974; Turnbull, 1974). Researchers concluded that a primary reason for short-term memory deficits was inefficient rehearsal activities. Apparently, the individuals with intellectual disability had the capability of rehearsing fairly efficiently, but they did not do so spontaneously (see Bray and Turner, 1986; Brown, 1974; Brown, Campione and Murphy, 1974).

By the early 1990s it was becoming clear that individuals with Down syndrome had a specific type of 'short-term memory' deficit, related to aurally presented verbal material, and more severe in magnitude than in unknown etiology groups (the phonological working memory difficulty discussed in the first part of this chapter). Thus, training studies specific to individuals with Down syndrome began to take place. Most of these training studies used the same basic training technique as the earlier training studies involving nonspecific etiology. This technique was overt cumulative rehearsal, which requires the participant to repeat back items aloud from the beginning of the list each time a new item is presented. This appeared to approximate the type of rehearsal individuals without intellectual disability were doing spontaneously in early studies. For example, if the sequence of items is *car, ball, dog,* the examiner would give *car* first and the participant would repeat *car.* Then the examiner would give *ball* and the participant would repeat *car, ball.* Finally, the examiner would give *dog* and the participant would repeat *car, ball, dog.*

Studies using overt cumulative rehearsal with individuals with Down syndrome have shown that training can indeed improve performance on working memory tasks. For example, Broadley and MacDonald (1993) found that two 20-minute rehearsal training sessions per week over six weeks resulted in increases in visual word span. Also, Comblain (1994) found that one 30-minute rehearsal training session per week over eight weeks improved phonological memory span. Laws, MacDonald and Buckley (1996) also reported gains in some phonological working memory measures after three 15-minute rehearsal training sessions per week over six weeks. Though few in number, these studies can be used to guide the development of interventions targeting phonological working memory. In the present section I describe the training routines used in these studies and I discuss the impact of the training. Finally, I suggest that, as researchers learn more about exactly what gives rise to phonological working memory difficulties in Down syndrome, training techniques other than, or complementary to, overt cumulative rehearsal may be warranted.

Nature of the training

Broadley and MacDonald's (1993) study involved two types of memory training – overt cumulative rehearsal and organization training. Half the training group began with six weeks of rehearsal training and continued with six weeks of organization training. The other half began with organization training and continued with rehearsal training. In the present chapter, the focus is on the rehearsal training, which is described in detail by Broadley (1994).

In this study, the six weeks of rehearsal training began with verbal labelling practice. The researcher showed pictures of common objects, one at a time, and asked the participant to name each picture aloud and repeat the name aloud. Next, an induced verbal rehearsal stage began in which the researcher taught the participant how to cumulatively rehearse more than one item. The researcher showed the first picture in a sequence and asked the participant to name it aloud. Then the researcher showed the second picture, and asked the participant to name both the first and second pictures aloud. When the participant hesitated or said the wrong name, the researcher prompted the participant by pointing and saying the picture. The next stage was cumulative rehearsal, in which the participant cumulatively rehearsed up to six items depending on his or her memory span. The researcher laid out pictures from left to right, in windows that could be opened one at a time to reveal a picture. The researcher opened the first window and named the picture, the participant repeated the name, and the researcher closed the window. The researcher asked the participant to recall the picture and then opened the window to reveal the picture for feedback. For sequences of two or more this procedure was repeated, always starting from the first window.

Laws et al. (1996) used a close variant of this procedure, though the method of displaying the pictures was modified to be more portable. The pictures in this study were from five categories and corresponded to one-, two-, and three-syllable words.

Comblain's (1994) rehearsal training took place in 30-minute sessions once a week over eight weeks. Each session was slightly different from the previous one, although the general procedure was the same throughout the eight sessions. Pictures were used in the first four sessions. The researcher showed a picture, named it and asked the participant to repeat the item. Then the researcher turned the picture over and asked the participant to recall it. If recall was correct, the researcher showed a second picture, named it, asked the participant to repeat the name, and turned it over. This time, the researcher asked the participant to recall both pictures, beginning with the first one. The procedure continued in this way, with recall always beginning from the first picture.

In the first session, only pictures from the same semantic category were used and the researcher presented pictures from the beginning each time a new item was added. In the second session, pictures from different semantic categories were used, again with pictures presented from the beginning each time. Next, pictures from the same semantic category were used, but this time the researcher did not present the pictures from the beginning each time. Instead, the researcher simply presented the next picture and the participant was to repeat from the beginning without the overt prompt. The fourth session was similar to the third, except that pictures were from different categories. Sessions five to eight followed the same sequence as sessions one to four except that instead of showing pictures and naming them, the researcher simply said the words aloud. To help the participant remember how many words there were, the researcher raised one finger each time he or she said a new word.

Impact of the training

Although there are only a few rehearsal training studies to draw upon, we can begin to look at the emerging patterns of the impact of the training on phonological working memory and on other cognitive functions. To evaluate the scope of the impact of the training, it is important to bear in mind the type of comparison each study makes. Laws et al. (1996) used a pretest–posttest design with no control group. In this design, significant gains are probably meaningful most of the time, but some degree of improvement over the time period of the training may be due to maturation or testing effects. The addition of a control group helps rule out these explanations. Comblain (1994) included both a trained group and an untrained control group, and could compare gains in the trained group to gains in the untrained control group. Still, some improvement may be due to increased compliance, motivation, or communication related to meeting with the researcher multiple times. An even more rigorous design is one that includes an active control group that meets with the researcher as often as the training group does, and so has the same amount of experience with the researcher. If the training group improves more than the active control group, it is likely that the improvements are due to the training and little else. Broadley and MacDonald's (1993) design, though perhaps not conceived in this way, can be used as such. Gains in the rehearsal training group can be compared not only with the untrained control group, but also with the organization training group, which is an active control group that did not have rehearsal training. Thus, in the discussion that follows, I evaluate the range of gains in light of the rigour of the design of each study.

In each of the three studies, rehearsal training involved words. All three studies began their training using pictures to represent words. Laws et al. (1996) and Broadley and MacDonald (1993) used pictures throughout, whereas Comblain (1994) phased out pictures to end training with spoken words. Across all studies, word-span tasks showed clear improvement. They showed improvement from pretest to posttest (Laws et al., 1996), greater improvement in the rehearsal-trained group than in the control group (Comblain, 1994), and greater improvement in the rehearsal trained group than in the active control group (Broadley and MacDonald, 1993). The word-span improvements were clear, however, only for measures of word span that were most similar to the training. When training phased out picture cues, ending with only auditory stimuli, there were improvements in auditory span (Comblain, 1994). When picture cues were used throughout the training, there were improvements in visual span but limited improvements in auditory span (Broadley and MacDonald, 1993; Laws et al., 1996). Specifically, the effects of training on word span generalized across modality (from visual to auditory) in the pre–posttest comparison of Laws, et al. (1996), but generally not in the active control group comparison of Broadley and MacDonald (1993). The effects did not generalize to digit span (presented visually or aurally) or nonword repetition (Laws et al., 1996). There was significant improvement in sentence memory from pretest to posttest (Laws, et al., 1996) but no difference in improvement between rehearsal-trained and active control groups (Broadley and MacDonald, 1993).

Thus, unless the training required participants to process auditory stimuli without picture cues (Comblain's study only), there was only weak evidence of improvement in phonological working memory. The effects of the picture-cued rehearsal training, however, did not necessarily generalize to picture memory either, though. There was no difference between rehearsal-trained and active control groups in picture memory (Broadley and MacDonald, 1993), although groups that had both rehearsal training and organization training had better picture memory following training than the untrained control group. Improvements seemed to be best on tasks that were very similar to the training routine in each study.

Thus, for assessments immediately following training, the range of cognitive functions enhanced by rehearsal training appears to be limited. Further, the rehearsal training in these studies was not necessarily effective for all participants. Comblain (1994) reported that, although pretest–posttest gains were significant for the children and adolescents in the study, they were not significant for the adults. Laws et al. (1996) reported that, although children trained by teachers and teaching assistants improved significantly from pretest to posttest, those trained by parents did not. Follow-up assessments indicate that improvements in modality-specific word span measures persist for at least eight months following completion of training (Comblain, 1994; Broadley, MacDonald and Buckley, 1994), but they are lost by three years following training (Laws et al., 1995). Improvements in related measures did not emerge over the follow-up period (Broadley et al., 1994; Laws, et al., 1995).

From the training studies, then, we know that it is possible to increase phonological working memory with rehearsal training, but perhaps only if the training specifically requires direct phonological processing (see Conners, Rosenquist and Taylor, in press). We do not know whether an increase in phonological working memory can boost language processing or other higher-order cognitive skills. Thus there is still much work to do on how to make memory training more effective for individuals with Down syndrome. This work should involve, first and foremost, an examination of the nature of the phonological working memory difficulty in Down syndrome. Once this difficulty is better understood, more effective interventions can be designed and tested. Thus, I turn next to the evidence that has begun to piece apart the specific relative weakness in phonological working memory.

What exactly is wrong with phonological working memory?

Baddeley's model can be used as a framework for looking for the locus or loci of the phonological working memory difficulty in Down syndrome. In this model (Baddeley, 1986; Baddeley and Hitch, 1974; 1994), phonological working memory consists of two components – the phonological store and the rehearsal loop. The phonological store holds speech-coded information for up to two seconds, after which the information would decay if not refreshed by the rehearsal loop. The rehearsal loop refreshes the information by repeatedly replaying it in a speech-like way. According to the model, if information is stored in a speech-like code, it should be more difficult to recall phonologically similar items than phonologically distinct items because they should be more confusable (phonological similarity effect). Also, according to the model, if information is refreshed in a subarticulatory rehearsal loop, there should be a relation between the time it takes to overtly articulate items and difficulty of recall. Items that take longer to articulate should be harder to recall because they are not rehearsed as many times in the same span of time (word-length effect). These basic effects have been examined in individuals with Down syndrome, but there are also other data that might help to pinpoint the locus of the phonological working memory difficulty in Down syndrome.

The rehearsal loop

One possibility for a locus of the phonological working memory difficulty is failure to rehearse. A failure to rehearse has been identified in other groups with intellectual disability, and cumulative rehearsal training has been the preferred memory-training technique to date for individuals with Down syndrome (but see Farb and Throne, 1978; Broadley and MacDonald, 1993).

The strongest case for a rehearsal problem in individuals with Down syndrome was made by Hulme and Mackenzie (1992), who found no word-length effect in participants with Down syndrome and both slower articulation speed and flatter slopes of recall over speech rate in participants with Down syndrome than in typically developing children. The absence of word-length effect suggested that participants with Down syndrome were not engaging in subarticulatory rehearsal; otherwise longer words would have been more difficult than shorter words. The slower articulation rate suggested that individuals with Down syndrome were limited in how fast they could recycle phonological codes. The flatter slopes of recall over speech rate suggested that recall was not related to articulation in the same way in participants with Down syndrome. Hulme and Mackenzie made a compelling case, but their study did not replicate the specific weakness in phonological working memory related to Down syndrome, and in fact showed no differences between Downs and intellectual disability groups. Although participants with DS performed worse on auditory span than typically developing children, they were no worse than participants with intellectual disability. Thus, the failure to rehearse they observed was not specific to Down syndrome and cannot account for the specific weakness in phonological working memory.

Jarrold et al. (2000) also demonstrated that, whereas individuals with Down syndrome may not rehearse efficiently, failure to rehearse cannot account for their poor word span performance. In experiment 1, participants with Down syndrome and participants with intellectual disability recalled lists consisting of long and short spoken words. The group with Down syndrome performed worse overall, but both groups showed significant word-length effects of equal magnitude. This suggested that both groups were rehearsing to the same degree, yet they differed in auditory span. Thus, rehearsal inefficiency could not account for the poor auditory span performance in the group with Down syndrome. However, because participants gave their responses orally, it was possible that the word-length effect was due to articulatory readout rather than rehearsal per se. Long words may have been more difficult to remember because they take longer to report, and so must be remembered over a longer span of time compared to short words. Thus, in experiment 2 the researchers examined word length effects using a probed recall task, which minimized articulatory readout. The word-length effects disappeared for the group with Down syndrome as well as for intellectual disability and typically developing groups, and the authors concluded that it was likely that none of the groups was rehearsing systematically. Yet, the group with Down syndrome still performed worse than the other groups at recalling the first-presented stimulus. The authors' general conclusion was that, whereas individuals with Down syndrome may not rehearse, failure to rehearse is not the cause of their phonological working memory difficulty.

Phonological store

Perhaps the first question to ask in regard to the phonological store is whether individuals with Down syndrome use speech-based codes in auditory span tasks. If so, they should show a phonological similarity effect in which similar-sounding words are more difficult to recall than different-sounding words. Indeed, several authors have reported significant phonological similarity effects in individuals with Down syndrome (Broadley et al., 1995; Hulme and Mackenzie, 1992; Jarrold et al., 2000). When the size of the effect was compared to that of intellectual disability or typically developing individuals, results were mixed. Jarrold et al. (2000) reported equivalent phonological similarity effects for their group with Down syndrome as for their intellectual disability and typically developing groups. Hulme and Mackenzie (1992) reported equivalent effects for groups with Down syndrome and intellectual disability but a larger effect in the typically developing group. Varnhagan et al. (1987) reported a significant effect only in the intellectual disability group and not in the group with Down syndrome. It should be noted that, in the latter two studies, the specific phonological working memory deficit was not replicated. Thus, most of the available evidence suggests that individuals with Down syndrome use phonological codes. Whether they use them as efficiently as other individuals with intellectual disability is not yet clear.

One index of the efficiency of phonological coding in working memory is the ease with which phonological codes in long-term memory can be accessed. As a person listens to a word, the first sounds in the speech signal activate candidate words in long-term memory, and often the word is identified before it is completely spoken (see Grosjean, 1980; Salasoo and Pisoni, 1985). If codes in long-term memory help to identify the word, they also help to specify the phonological code in working memory. Varnhagan et al. (1987) suggested that individuals with Down syndrome have poor access to phonological codes in long-term memory. They found that participants with Down syndrome were equivalent on many measures to matched participants with intellectual disability, however, they were worse on a task that measured speed of retrieval of phonological codes from long-term memory. This was the Posner letter-matching task, in which participants say, as quickly as possible, whether or not two letters match physically (for example, BB, BA), and whether or not two letters share the same name (for example, Bb, Ba). Speed of physical matching is subtracted from speed of name matching to yield a measure of access to phonological codes in long-term memory. As noted previously, Varnhagan et al. (1987) did not replicate the specific phonological working memory weakness in Down syndrome, so interpretation of other effects are difficult. However, lexical access measures correlated with verbal span measures in the DS group only. Also, other studies provide evidence consistent with this idea.

Marcell and Cohen (1992) replicated the phonological working memory weakness in Down syndrome by showing that participants with Down syndrome performed more poorly than matched participants with intellectual disability on auditory digit span as well as sentence imitation. Participants with Down syndrome also performed more poorly than participants with intellectual disability group on two tasks that required retrieval of phonological codes from long-term memory. One was a gating task in which only portions of the auditory signal of words were played, and participants guessed what the word was. Participants with Down syndrome needed to hear a greater percentage of the word to make a correct identification, compared with the intellectual disability group. The other was a masked word identification task, in which a spoken word was followed by a sound mask 40 ms after presentation. Although the participants with Down syndrome did no worse than those with intellectual disability when the mask was delayed, they did worse when the mask came 40 ms after the word. One interpretation is that they were slower than participants with intellectual disability at accessing the phonological code in long-term memory. At 40 ms after the presentation of the word, they still had not completely accessed many of the words and as a result made mistakes. Although measures of hearing (speech reception threshold and tympanic reflex but not pure tone threshold) correlated with this measure, they did not correlate with the digit span, sentence memory, or gating task measures.

Two other findings are consistent with inefficient access to phonological codes in long-term memory, although they could be interpreted in other ways as well. In one study, typically developing comparison groups had longer auditory spans for fast-presented items than for slow-presented items, but participants with Down syndrome were not affected by rate of item presentation (Marcell and Armstrong, 1982). If access to phonological codes were slow or otherwise inefficient in Down syndrome, more time would be needed to code each item as it is presented; thus the advantage for fast-presented items would be lost.

In another study, participants with Down syndrome were slower than participants with intellectual disability and typically developing participants to initiate responses for phonological memory tasks (sentence memory), but not for other oral-verbal tasks (Marcell, Ridgeway, Sewell and Whelan, 1995). This effect was present only on the sentence imitation task, so it could not be interpreted as a general speed-related problem in preparing and initiating responses. Instead, the authors suggest that encoding of phonological information requires so many cognitive resources for individuals with Down syndrome, few are available for response preparation. Thus, the result of inefficient phonological coding is slowed response preparation only in tasks requiring phonological coding. As suggested previously, phonological coding involves access of phonological codes from long-term memory. These results and the others just discussed suggest that researchers should look more closely at phonological codes in individuals with Down syndrome.

The next phase of intervention research

In the best possible world, interventions would be designed with a full understanding of the problem at hand. In the real world, however, needs are apparent, and we design interventions that make sense and might work, without always having that full understanding. This is what has happened in the case of phonological working memory training for individuals with Down syndrome. The interventions that have been tried have led to improvements, but the improvements have been fairly limited both in range of cognitive functions affected and in longevity. Yet, it is clear that at least limited improvements are possible using overt cumulative rehearsal. That fact is extremely important because it encourages the next phase of intervention research.

The next phase should begin with intense research on the nature of the phonological working memory deficit in Down syndrome. This will involve examining rehearsal processes as well as phonological coding and storage processes. Although the present evidence regarding rehearsal processes suggests that any failure to rehearse is not directly responsible for the phonological working memory deficit (see Jarrold et al., 2000 for a discussion), there is still very little evidence to bring to bear on this question. Replications are needed, using different methods for measuring rehearsal. The existing evidence regarding phonological coding suggests that individuals with Down syndrome use phonological codes in memory span tasks, but many questions still remain concerning, for example, the quality and durability of phonological codes in working memory and the quantity of phonological information that can be stored in working memory at one time. Some of the current evidence suggests an inefficiency of access to phonological codes in long-term memory. Will further evidence confirm this hypothesis? If so, is this a problem of access per se, or the quality of phonological representations in long-term memory?

Even though we do not fully understand the nature of the phonological working memory deficit, it is plain that two elements should be incorporated into the next set of interventions. The first is cumulative rehearsal, because it can boost immediate memory. Even if failure to rehearse is not the reason for such difficulty with phonological working memory, keeping more information active at a given time can enable other key memory functions. Researchers should examine the parameters of rehearsal techniques to determine how they can be made more efficient. The second element that should be incorporated into the next set

agan S (1987) Auditory and visual memory span: co
MR individuals with Down syndrome and oth
nal of Mental Deficiency 91: 398–405.
agirone C (1995) Short-term memory in persons wit
d Down's syndrome. Journal of Intellectual Disabilit

hological profile of Down syndrome: cognitive skill
ental Retardation and Developmental Disabilitie

idence from two genetic syndromes for a dissoci
sual-spatial short-term memory. Journal of Clinical
chology 16: 317–22.

of interventions is practice in basic phonological processes such as discrimination and identification. Given the possibility that access to phonological codes in long-term memory is inefficient in individuals with Down syndrome, practice that involves both newly encountered codes and codes stored in long-term memory would be advisable.

Acknowledgement

Preparation of this chapter was supported by Grant HD37445 from the National Institute of Child Health and Human Development, jointly with the National Down Syndrome Society.

References

Baddeley, AD (1986) Working memory. Oxford: Oxford University Press.
Baddeley AD, Hitch G (1974). Working memory. In GH Bower (ed.) Recent Advances in Learning and Motivation. New York: Academic Press, vol. 8, pp. 47–89.
Baddeley AD, Hitch G (1994) Developments in the concept of working memory. Neuropsychology 8: 485–93.
Belmont JM, Butterfield EC (1969) The relations of short-term memory to development and intelligence. In LP Lipsett, HW Reese (eds) Advances in Child Development and Behavior. New York: Academic Press, vol. 4, pp. 29–82.
Bilovsky D, Share J (1965) The ITPA and Down's syndrome: an exploratory study. American Journal of Mental Deficiency 70: 78–82.
Bower A, Hayes A (1994) Short-term memory deficits and Down syndrome: a comparative study. Down Syndrome Research and Practice 2: 47–50.
Bray NW, Turner LA (1986) The rehearsal deficit hypothesis. In NR Ellis, NW Bray (eds) International Review of Research in Mental Retardation. New York: Academic Press, vol. 14, pp. 47–71.
Broadley I (1994) Teaching short term memory skills to children with Down's syndrome. Unpublished dissertation, University of Portsmouth, Portsmouth, England.
Broadley I, MacDonald J (1993) Teaching short-term memory skills to children with Down syndrome. Down Syndrome Research and Practice 1: 56–62.
Broadley I, MacDonald J, Buckley S (1994) Are children with Down syndrome able to maintain skills learned from a short-term memory training program? Down Syndrome Research and Practice 2: 116–22.
Broadley I, MacDonald J, Buckley S (1995) Working memory in children with Down syndrome. Down Syndrome Research and Practice 3: 3–8.
Brown AL (1974) The role of strategic behavior in retardate memory. In NR Ellis (ed.) International Review of Research in Mental Retardation. New York: Academic Press, vol. 7, pp. 55–111.
Brown AL, Campione JC, Bray NW, Wilcox BL (1973) Keeping track of changing variables: Effects of rehearsal training and rehearsal prevention in normal and retarded adolescents. Journal of Experimental Psychology 101: 123–31.
Brown AL, Campione JC, Murphy MD (1974) Keeping track of changing variables: long-term retention of a trained rehearsal strategy by retarded adolescents. American Journal of Mental Deficiency 78: 446–53.

Burr DB, Rohr A (1978) Patterns of psycholinguistic development in the severely mentally retarded: a hypothesis. Social Biology 25: 15–22.

Chapman RS, Hesketh LJ (2000) Behavioral phenotype of individuals with Down syndrome. Mental Retardation and Developmental Disabilities Research Reviews 6: 84–95.

Comblain A (1994) Working memory in Down syndrome: training the rehearsal strategy. Down Syndrome Research and Practice 2: 123–6.

Conners FA, Rosenquist CJ, Taylor LA (in press) Memory training for children with Down syndrome. Down Syndrome Research and Practice.

Conroy RL (1978) Facilitation of serial recall in retarded children and adolescents: verbal and kinesthetic strategies. American Journal of Mental Deficiency 82: 410–13.

Crowe SF, Hay DA (1990) Neuropsychological dimensions of the fragile X syndrome: support for a non-dominant hemisphere dysfunction hypothesis. Neuropsychologia 28: 9–16.

Ellis NR (1970) Memory processes in retardates and normals: theoretical and empirical considerations. In NR Ellis (ed.) International review of research in mental retardation. New York: Academic Press, vol. 4, pp. 1–32.

Farb J, Throne JM (1978) Improving the generalized mnemonic performance of a Down's syndrome child. Journal of Applied Behavior Analysis 11: 413–19.

Gathercole SE,, Baddeley AD (1993) Working memory and language. Hillsdale NJ: Lawrence Erlbaum Associates.

Grosjean F (1980) Spoken word recognition processes and the gating paradigm. Perception and Psychophysics 28: 267–83.

Hitch GJ, Woodin ME, Baker S (1989) Visual and phonological components of working memory in children. Memory and Cognition 17: 175–85.

Hitch GJ, Halliday S, Schaafstal AM, Schraagen JML (1988) Visual working memory in young children. Memory and Cognition 16: 120–32.

Hulme C, Mackenzie S (1992) Working memory and severe learning difficulties. Hillsdale NJ: Lawrence Erlbaum Associates.

Jarrold C, Baddeley AD (1997) Short-term memory for verbal and visuo-spatial information in Down's syndrome. Cognitive Neuropsychiatry 2: 101–22.

Jarrold C, Baddeley AD, Hewes AK (1999) Genetically dissociated components working memory: evidence from Down's and Williams syndro Neuropsychologia 37: 637–51.

Jarrold C, Baddeley AD, Hewes AK (2000) Verbal short-term memory defic Down syndrome: a consequence of problems in rehearsal? Journal of Psychology and Psychiatry 40: 233–44.

Jarrold C, Baddeley AD, Phillips C (1999) Down syndrome and the phono loop: the evidence for, and importance of, a specific verbal short-term deficit. Down Syndrome Research and Practice 6: 61–75.

Kay-Raining Bird E, Chapman RS (1994) Sequential recall in individ Down syndrome. Journal of Speech and Hearing Research 37:1369–

Kellas G, Ashcraft MH, Johnson NS (1974) Rehearsal processes in the memory performance of mildly retarded adolescents. American Mental Deficiency 77: 670–9.

Klein BP, Mervis CB (1999) Contrasting patterns of cognitive abilities year-olds with Williams syndrome or Down syndrome. Dev Neuropsychology 16: 177–96.

Laws G (19
   childrer
   1119–

Laws G,
   a reh
   synd

Laws C
   me
   Re

Mack
   s

Ma

Varnhagan CK, Das JP, Va
   nitive processing by
   etiologies. American Jou

Vicari S, Carlesimo GA, Calt
   intellectual disabilities an
   Research 39: 532–7.

Wang PP (1996) A neuropsyc
   and brain morphology. M
   Research Reviews 2: 102–8

Wang PP, Bellugi U (1994) Ev
   ation between verbal and v
   and Experimental Neuropsy

Chapter 4
Speech acquisition and approaches to intervention

CAROL STOEL-GAMMON

Introduction

The acquisition of speech and language is one of the most remarkable feats of childhood. Children begin to produce words around their first birthday, can create short sentences by their second birthday and, by the age of 8, have a good command of the phonological and syntactic properties of their mother tongue. There are, however, groups of children who, for one reason or another, fail to acquire spoken language in the same fashion as typically developing children. Speech and language disorders can stem from a variety of factors, including hearing loss, orofacial anomalies, and cognitive impairment. Individually, each of these factors is likely to have a negative impact the acquisition of speech and language. Presence of more than one factor creates an even greater impact. Speech development of children with Down syndrome is clearly affected by these factors, though the exact influences, singly or in combination, are difficult to determine. Even when matched for mental age, children with Down syndrome lag behind non-Down syndrome peers in the acquisition of speech and language (Miller, 1988).

The goal of this chapter is twofold: to provide an overview of speech development in children with Down syndrome and to discuss approaches to intervention for these children. The overview and discussion of intervention focus on four aspects of speech development: factors that create difficulties with speech acquisition; pre-speech patterns and first words; the phonology of single words; and intelligibility. It should be noted at the outset that, although general statements are made throughout this chapter, individuals with Down syndrome exhibit a wide range of speech and language abilities; thus, the generalizations presented will not necessarily hold true for all children.

Contributing factors

Anatomical and structural differences

Children with Down syndrome differ from typically developing children on a variety of anatomical and physiological features associated with speech production. These features include differences in the vocal cords, presence of a high palatal vault, a larger than typical tongue in relation to the oral cavity, weak facial muscles, and general hypotonicity (Leddy, 1999; Miller and Leddy, 1998; Rast and Harris, 1985). Although the precise effect of these differences is difficult to determine, they undoubtedly influence the development of articulatory and phonatory abilities.

The nervous system of individuals with Down syndrome also has distinctive characteristics, including anatomical differences in the central and peripheral nervous system, reduced brain size and weight, smaller and fewer sulci, narrower superior temporal gyrus, fewer cortical neurons, decreased neuronal density, delayed neuronal myelination; abnormal dendrite structures; and altered cellular membranes (Leddy, 1999; Miller, 1988; Miller and Leddy, 1998). These differences appear to be associated with disruptions in the accuracy, speed, consistency and economy of speech movements, and thus have a direct influence on the production of speech.

Hearing status

An additional factor for children with Down syndrome is fluctuating hearing loss associated with otitis media and middle-ear pathologies (Balkany, 1980). Downs (1980) reported that 78% of the children she assessed had a 15 dB loss, or greater, in one or both ears; 65% of these displayed significant levels of loss in both ears. Greater degrees of loss and/or extended periods of middle ear disease are likely to be associated with poorer outcomes on speech and language. This conclusion is supported by Chapman (1997) who noted that much of the variation in communicative abilities of individuals with Down syndrome is better understood when hearing status is taken into account.

Summary

Children with Down syndrome differ from peers with typical development on a variety of factors: cognitive level, anatomy and physiology of structures involved in speech production, and hearing status. Taken together, these factors undoubtedly have strong influences on the acquisition of speech and language.

Pre-speech and early speech development

Typical developmental patterns

The foundations for speech development occur in the first year of life with the emergence of vocalizations that serve as precursors for the production of words and phrases. Of particular importance to later speech development is the use of consonant-vowel syllables, such as [baba], which generally appear around 6 to 7 months (Oller, 1980). Phonetically, these 'canonical' babbles are similar, or even identical, to forms used in first words; thus, the phonetic form [mama] may be a non-meaningful babble at 8 months and a word at 14 months. The difference is awareness that words are based on an arbitrary relationship between sound and meaning. The timetable for development of babble and emergence of words is well documented, and is stable across socio-economic classes and different language environments. Hearing impairment, however, has been shown to cause substantial delays in the onset of canonical babble (Oller and Eilers, 1988; Stoel-Gammon and Otomo, 1986) and in the production of words.

In a typically developing child, first words appear around the end of the first year, overlapping with the period of late canonical babble; thereafter, babble and speech coexist for many months. When children have a productive vocabulary of about 10 different words, the proportion of words and babble in their spontaneous productions is roughly equal (Robb, Bauer and Tyler, 1994). When the productive vocabulary reaches 50 words, at around 18 months, the ratio of words to babble is about three to one.

During the transition to words, the phonetic characteristics of babble and speech are highly similar. Specifically, consonants that occur most frequently in babbling (stops, nasals, glides) also predominate in early word productions, while consonants that are infrequent in babble (fricatives, affricates, liquids) are precisely those that are acquired late in meaningful speech. Moreover, the consonant–vowel syllable structure, characteristic of canonical babbling period, is the most frequent syllabic type in early word productions. Thus, babbling and early speech share the same basic phonetic properties in terms of sound types and syllable structures (Stoel-Gammon, 1998).

There is a growing body of evidence linking pre-speech vocal development with general speech and language skills throughout early childhood (Stoel-Gammon, 1992). In general, increased use of complex babble in the prelinguistic period is linked to better performance on the speech and language measures after the onset of speech. Stoel-Gammon (1998) hypothesized that infants who produce more babble, particularly more canonical utterances with a variety of consonants and vowels, exhibit better early language skills because they have amassed a greater arsenal of 'building blocks' that can be recruited for the production of a wide variety of words.

Effects of Down syndrome

Although children with Down syndrome are delayed in the acquisition of speech and language skills, investigations of pre-speech development suggest that they are nearly typical in this domain. Dodd (1972) compared the babbling patterns of 10 infants with Down syndrome, and 10 typically developing infants. Despite differences on measures of mental and motor development, analyses of 15-minute recordings of spontaneous vocalizations revealed no significant differences between the two groups in terms of number of utterances, length of utterances, time spent vocalizing, and variety of consonant and vowel sounds produced. Dodd concluded that babbling does not reflect intelligence at this stage of development. Smith and Oller (1981) compared infants with Down syndrome with typically developing peers and reported similarities in age of onset of reduplicated canonical babble, place of articulation of consonants, and vowel quality. Longitudinal studies by Steffens, Oller, Lynch and Urbano (1992) and Smith and Stoel-Gammon (1996) also revealed that pre-speech patterns of infants with Down syndrome closely resemble those of typically developing peers.

In contrast to the studies cited above, Lynch and colleagues (Lynch, Oller, Steffens, Levine, Basinger, and Umbel, 1995) reported two differences in a longitudinal investigation of 13 infants with Down syndrome and 27 typically developing infants. First, the average age of onset of canonical babbling among the infants with Down syndrome was about 9 months, approximately two months later than the age for the typically developing infants. Second, over time, the occurrence of canonical babbling was less stable for the infants with Down syndrome. Hypotonicity and delays in motor development are characteristic of Down syndrome, so the relative instability in canonical babbling may be a consequence of deficits in the motor domain. These findings notwithstanding, it appears that Down syndrome has relatively little effect on pre-speech vocal development. In large measure, developmental patterns are within typical range, although the pre-speech period is much longer, often extending through the second year of life.

In contrast to the findings regarding pre-speech development, children with Down syndrome exhibit a substantial delay in the transition to meaningful speech and, once words appear, are slow to build an expressive vocabulary. Stray-Gunderson (1986) reported that some children produced words as early as 9 months (chronological age), within the range for children with typical development; for other children, first words did not appear until the age of 7. On average, however, word production was delayed. Buckley (2000) reported that the average productive vocabulary for 24-month-old children in her group with Down syndrome was 28 (compared with 250 for a typically developing child). At 3 years, the mean vocabulary was 116 words, rising to 248 words at 4 years, and to 330 words at 6 years, an age at which the child with typically development has a vocabulary of several thousand words. Other investigations of lexical acquisition in children with Down syndrome have shown that even when they are matched to a typically developing comparison group on mental (rather than chronological) age, lexical acquisition in children with Down syndrome is delayed (Chapman, 1997).

Single-word phonology

Typical developmental patterns

Phonological acquisition of children with typical development has been well documented. In the early stages, words are 'simplified' in terms of their structure: consonant clusters are reduced to single consonants, unstressed syllables are deleted, and consonants at the ends of words may be omitted. In terms of consonantal classes, stops, nasals and glides are generally acquired early, while fricatives, affricates and liquids are mastered later. Correct production of most vowels is achieved by 4 years (Stoel-Gammon and Herrington, 1990). Among children acquiring English, correct pronunciation of all phonemes is achieved by the age of 8 (Sander, 1972).

Effects of Down syndrome

A number of investigations of speech and language of individuals with mental retardation have reported that articulatory/phonological problems are particularly severe for children with Down syndrome (Blanchard 1968; Dodd 1975, 1976; Dodd and Leahy, 1989; Rosenberg and Abbeduto, 1993; Stoel-Gammon 1981). Production errors of these children resemble errors that occur in typical phonological development: fricatives, affricates and liquids have higher rates of error than stop, nasal and glide consonants (Bleile and Schwarz, 1984; Mackay and Hodson, 1982; Smith and Stoel-Gammon, 1983; Stoel-Gammon, 1981).

Analyses of error patterns (phonological processes) have also highlighted similarities between children with Down syndrome and those with typical development; in both groups, the following patterns are present:

* consonant clusters are produced as singleton consonants
* word-final consonants are omitted
* target fricatives and affricates are produced as stops
* aspirated voiceless stops in initial position are deaspirated
* word-initial liquids are produced as glides
* word-final liquids are produced as vowels or are omitted, and
* word-final voiced obstruents are devoiced (Bleiele and Schwarz, 1984; Cholmain, 1994; Dodd, 1976; Kumin, Councill and Goodman, 1994; Mackay and Hodson, 1982; Smith and Stoel-Gammon, 1983; Stoel-Gammon, 1980; Van Borsel, 1996).

Despite the similarities across groups, differences are also evident. Perhaps the most striking is rate of development. As might be expected, phonological development among children with Down syndrome proceeds at a slower rate than in their cognitively typical peers (Smith and Stoel-Gammon, 1983) and errors documented for young children with Down syndrome tend to persist through adolescence and into adulthood (Shriberg and Widder, 1990; Sommers, Reinhart and Sistrunk, 1988; Sommers, Patterson, and Wildgen, 1988).

In addition, the speech of children with Down syndrome exhibits more variability and a higher proportion of 'non-developmental' error types. Dodd (1976) compared the phonological systems of three groups of children matched for mental age: typical, intellectual disabled, and Down syndrome. The performance of children in the Down syndrome group differed from the other groups in several aspects. They made a greater number of phonological errors in their productions; their errors were more inconsistent; and a greater proportion of their errors could not be described by a set of common phonological processes. Stoel-Gammon (1981) also reported greater variability in errors, noting that children with typical development move from incorrect to correct phoneme production in a linear fashion with a small set of substitution types. In contrast, among children with Down syndrome, there was a greater range of substitution types and greater variation in errors from one word to another.

Intelligibility

Typical developmental patterns

Intelligibility (the degree to which speech can be understood) is influenced by a variety of causes, and the relationship between intelligibility and phonological skills is not straightforward. Initially, young children are often unintelligible to all but their immediate family. Between the ages of 2 and 4 years, intelligibility increases dramatically: At 2 years, approximately half (50%) of a child's productions can be understood by an adult not familiar with the child; at 3 years the proportion of intelligible productions rises to 75%; and at 4 years, it reaches 100% (Coplan and Gleason, 1988). Of course, this does not mean that a 4-year-old has acquired all the elements of the phonological system; rather, that the types of errors that remain have little impact on level of intelligibility.

Effects of Down syndrome

Unintelligibility is one of the characteristics associated with Down syndrome, and the speech of many individuals with Down syndrome tends to be unintelligible throughout their lives even though their mental age may exceed 4 years (Kumin 1994; Pueschel and Hopman, 1993; Shriberg and Widder, 1990). Long-standing difficulties with intelligibility can of interventions is practice in basic phonological processes such as discrimination and identification. Given the possibility that access to phonological codes in long-term memory is inefficient in individuals with Down syndrome, practice that involves both newly encountered codes and codes stored in long-term memory would be advisable.

Acknowledgement

Preparation of this chapter was supported by Grant HD37445 from the National Institute of Child Health and Human Development, jointly with the National Down Syndrome Society.

References

Baddeley, AD (1986) Working memory. Oxford: Oxford University Press.

Baddeley AD, Hitch G (1974). Working memory. In GH Bower (ed.) Recent Advances in Learning and Motivation. New York: Academic Press, vol. 8, pp. 47–89.

Baddeley AD, Hitch G (1994) Developments in the concept of working memory. Neuropsychology 8: 485–93.

Belmont JM, Butterfield EC (1969) The relations of short-term memory to development and intelligence. In LP Lipsett, HW Reese (eds) Advances in Child Development and Behavior. New York: Academic Press, vol. 4, pp. 29–82.

Bilovsky D, Share J (1965) The ITPA and Down's syndrome: an exploratory study. American Journal of Mental Deficiency 70: 78–82.

Bower A, Hayes A (1994) Short-term memory deficits and Down syndrome: a comparative study. Down Syndrome Research and Practice 2: 47–50.

Bray NW, Turner LA (1986) The rehearsal deficit hypothesis. In NR Ellis, NW Bray (eds) International Review of Research in Mental Retardation. New York: Academic Press, vol. 14, pp. 47–71.

Broadley I (1994) Teaching short term memory skills to children with Down's syndrome. Unpublished dissertation, University of Portsmouth, Portsmouth, England.

Broadley I, MacDonald J (1993) Teaching short-term memory skills to children with Down syndrome. Down Syndrome Research and Practice 1: 56–62.

Broadley I, MacDonald J, Buckley S (1994) Are children with Down syndrome able to maintain skills learned from a short-term memory training program? Down Syndrome Research and Practice 2: 116–22.

Broadley I, MacDonald J, Buckley S (1995) Working memory in children with Down syndrome. Down Syndrome Research and Practice 3: 3–8.

Brown AL (1974) The role of strategic behavior in retardate memory. In NR Ellis (ed.) International Review of Research in Mental Retardation. New York: Academic Press, vol. 7, pp. 55–111.

Brown AL, Campione JC, Bray NW, Wilcox BL (1973) Keeping track of changing variables: Effects of rehearsal training and rehearsal prevention in normal and retarded adolescents. Journal of Experimental Psychology 101: 123–31.

Brown AL, Campione JC, Murphy MD (1974) Keeping track of changing variables: long-term retention of a trained rehearsal strategy by retarded adolescents. American Journal of Mental Deficiency 78: 446–53.

Burr DB, Rohr A (1978) Patterns of psycholinguistic development in the severely mentally retarded: a hypothesis. Social Biology 25: 15–22.

Chapman RS, Hesketh LJ (2000) Behavioral phenotype of individuals with Down syndrome. Mental Retardation and Developmental Disabilities Research Reviews 6: 84–95.

Comblain A (1994) Working memory in Down syndrome: training the rehearsal strategy. Down Syndrome Research and Practice 2: 123–6.

Conners FA, Rosenquist CJ, Taylor LA (in press) Memory training for children with Down syndrome. Down Syndrome Research and Practice.

Conroy RL (1978) Facilitation of serial recall in retarded children and adolescents: verbal and kinesthetic strategies. American Journal of Mental Deficiency 82: 410–13.

Crowe SF, Hay DA (1990) Neuropsychological dimensions of the fragile X syndrome: support for a non-dominant hemisphere dysfunction hypothesis. Neuropsychologia 28: 9–16.

Ellis NR (1970) Memory processes in retardates and normals: theoretical and empirical considerations. In NR Ellis (ed.) International review of research in mental retardation. New York: Academic Press, vol. 4, pp. 1–32.

Farb J, Throne JM (1978) Improving the generalized mnemonic performance of a Down's syndrome child. Journal of Applied Behavior Analysis 11: 413–19.

Gathercole SE,, Baddeley AD (1993) Working memory and language. Hillsdale NJ: Lawrence Erlbaum Associates.

Grosjean F (1980) Spoken word recognition processes and the gating paradigm. Perception and Psychophysics 28: 267–83.

Hitch GJ, Woodin ME, Baker S (1989) Visual and phonological components of working memory in children. Memory and Cognition 17: 175–85.

Hitch GJ, Halliday S, Schaafstal AM, Schraagen JML (1988) Visual working memory in young children. Memory and Cognition 16: 120–32.

Hulme C, Mackenzie S (1992) Working memory and severe learning difficulties. Hillsdale NJ: Lawrence Erlbaum Associates.

Jarrold C, Baddeley AD (1997) Short-term memory for verbal and visuo-spatial information in Down's syndrome. Cognitive Neuropsychiatry 2: 101–22.

Jarrold C, Baddeley AD, Hewes AK (1999) Genetically dissociated components of working memory: evidence from Down's and Williams syndrome. Neuropsychologia 37: 637–51.

Jarrold C, Baddeley AD, Hewes AK (2000) Verbal short-term memory deficits in Down syndrome: a consequence of problems in rehearsal? Journal of Child Psychology and Psychiatry 40: 233–44.

Jarrold C, Baddeley AD, Phillips C (1999) Down syndrome and the phonological loop: the evidence for, and importance of, a specific verbal short-term memory deficit. Down Syndrome Research and Practice 6: 61–75.

Kay-Raining Bird E, Chapman RS (1994) Sequential recall in individuals with Down syndrome. Journal of Speech and Hearing Research 37:1369–80.

Kellas G, Ashcraft MH, Johnson NS (1974) Rehearsal processes in the short-term memory performance of mildly retarded adolescents. American Journal of Mental Deficiency 77: 670–9.

Klein BP, Mervis CB (1999) Contrasting patterns of cognitive abilities of 9- and 10-year-olds with Williams syndrome or Down syndrome. Developmental Neuropsychology 16: 177–96.

Laws G (1998) The use of nonword repetition as a test of phonological memory in children with Down syndrome. Journal of Child Psychology and Psychiatry 39: 1119–30.

Laws G, MacDonald J, Buckley S (1996) The effects of a short training in the use of a rehearsal strategy on memory for words and pictures in children with Down syndrome. Down Syndrome Research and Practice 4: 70–8.

Laws G, MacDonald J, Buckley S, Broadley I (1995) Long-term maintenance of memory skills taught to children with Down syndrome. Down Syndrome Research and Practice 3: 103–9.

Mackenzie S, Hulme C (1987) Memory span development in Down's syndrome, severely subnormal and normal subjects. Cognitive Neuropsychology 4: 303–19.

Marcell MM, Armstrong V (1982) Auditory and visual sequential memory of Down syndrome and nonretarded children. American Journal of Mental Deficiency 87: 86–95.

Marcell MM, Cohen S (1992) Hearing abilities of Down syndrome and other mentally handicapped adolescents. Research in Developmental Disabilities 13: 533–51.

Marcell MM, Weeks SL (1988) Short-term memory difficulties and Down's syndrome. Journal of Mental Deficiency Research 32: 153–62.

Marcell MM, Ridgeway MM, Sewell DH, Whelan ML (1995) Sentence imitation by adolescents and young adults with Down's syndrome and other intellectual disabilities. Journal of Intellectual Disability Research 39: 215–32.

Marcell MM, Harvey CF, Cothran P (1988) An attempt to improve auditory short-term memory in Down's syndrome individuals through reducing distractions. Research in Developmental Disabilities 9: 405–17.

McDade HL, Adler S (1980) Down syndrome and short-term memory impairment: A storage or retrieval deficit? American Journal of Mental Deficiency 84: 561–7.

Prior MR (1977) Psycholinguistic disabilities of autistic and retarded children. Journal of Mental Deficiency Research 21: 37–45.

Pueschel SM, Gallagher PL, Zartler AS, Pezzullo JC (1987) Cognitive and learning processes in children with Down syndrome. Research in Developmental Disabilities 8: 21–37.

Rohr A, Burr DB (1978) Etiological differences in patterns of psycholinguistic development of children of IQ 30 to 60. American Journal of Mental Deficiency 82: 549–53.

Rondal JA, Lambert JL, Sohier C (1981) Elicited verbal and nonverbal imitation in Down's syndrome and other mentally retarded children: a replication and extension of Berry. Language and Speech 24: 245–54.

Salasoo A, Pisoni DB (1985) Interaction of knowledge sources in spoken word identification. Journal of Memory and Language 24: 210–31.

Schapiro MB, Murphy DGM, Hagerman RJ, Azari NP, Alexander GE, Miezejeski CM, Hinton VJ, Horowitz B, Haxby JV, Kumar A, White B, Grady CL (1995) Adult Fragile X syndrome: neuropsychology, brain anatomy, and metabolism. American Journal of Medical Genetics 60: 480–93.

Snart F, O'Grady M, Das JP (1982) Cognitive processing by subgroups of moderately mentally retarded children. American Journal of Mental Deficiency 86: 465–72.

Turnbull AP (1974) Teaching retarded persons to rehearse through cumulative overt labelling. American Journal of Mental Deficiency 79: 331–37.

Varnhagan CK, Das JP, Varnhagan S (1987) Auditory and visual memory span: cognitive processing by TMR individuals with Down syndrome and other etiologies. American Journal of Mental Deficiency 91: 398–405.

Vicari S, Carlesimo GA, Caltagirone C (1995) Short-term memory in persons with intellectual disabilities and Down's syndrome. Journal of Intellectual Disability Research 39: 532–7.

Wang PP (1996) A neuropsychological profile of Down syndrome: cognitive skills and brain morphology. Mental Retardation and Developmental Disabilities Research Reviews 2: 102–8.

Wang PP, Bellugi U (1994) Evidence from two genetic syndromes for a dissociation between verbal and visual-spatial short-term memory. Journal of Clinical and Experimental Neuropsychology 16: 317–22.

Chapter 4
Speech acquisition and approaches to intervention

CAROL STOEL-GAMMON

Introduction

The acquisition of speech and language is one of the most remarkable feats of childhood. Children begin to produce words around their first birthday, can create short sentences by their second birthday and, by the age of 8, have a good command of the phonological and syntactic properties of their mother tongue. There are, however, groups of children who, for one reason or another, fail to acquire spoken language in the same fashion as typically developing children. Speech and language disorders can stem from a variety of factors, including hearing loss, orofacial anomalies, and cognitive impairment. Individually, each of these factors is likely to have a negative impact the acquisition of speech and language. Presence of more than one factor creates an even greater impact. Speech development of children with Down syndrome is clearly affected by these factors, though the exact influences, singly or in combination, are difficult to determine. Even when matched for mental age, children with Down syndrome lag behind non-Down syndrome peers in the acquisition of speech and language (Miller, 1988).

The goal of this chapter is twofold: to provide an overview of speech development in children with Down syndrome and to discuss approaches to intervention for these children. The overview and discussion of intervention focus on four aspects of speech development: factors that create difficulties with speech acquisition; pre-speech patterns and first words; the phonology of single words; and intelligibility. It should be noted at the outset that, although general statements are made throughout this chapter, individuals with Down syndrome exhibit a wide range of speech and language abilities; thus, the generalizations presented will not necessarily hold true for all children.

49

Contributing factors

Anatomical and structural differences

Children with Down syndrome differ from typically developing children on a variety of anatomical and physiological features associated with speech production. These features include differences in the vocal cords, presence of a high palatal vault, a larger than typical tongue in relation to the oral cavity, weak facial muscles, and general hypotonicity (Leddy, 1999; Miller and Leddy, 1998; Rast and Harris, 1985). Although the precise effect of these differences is difficult to determine, they undoubtedly influence the development of articulatory and phonatory abilities.

The nervous system of individuals with Down syndrome also has distinctive characteristics, including anatomical differences in the central and peripheral nervous system, reduced brain size and weight, smaller and fewer sulci, narrower superior temporal gyrus, fewer cortical neurons, decreased neuronal density, delayed neuronal myelination; abnormal dendrite structures; and altered cellular membranes (Leddy, 1999; Miller, 1988; Miller and Leddy, 1998). These differences appear to be associated with disruptions in the accuracy, speed, consistency and economy of speech movements, and thus have a direct influence on the production of speech.

Hearing status

An additional factor for children with Down syndrome is fluctuating hearing loss associated with otitis media and middle-ear pathologies (Balkany, 1980). Downs (1980) reported that 78% of the children she assessed had a 15 dB loss, or greater, in one or both ears; 65% of these displayed significant levels of loss in both ears. Greater degrees of loss and/or extended periods of middle ear disease are likely to be associated with poorer outcomes on speech and language. This conclusion is supported by Chapman (1997) who noted that much of the variation in communicative abilities of individuals with Down syndrome is better understood when hearing status is taken into account.

Summary

Children with Down syndrome differ from peers with typical development on a variety of factors: cognitive level, anatomy and physiology of structures involved in speech production, and hearing status. Taken together, these factors undoubtedly have strong influences on the acquisition of speech and language.

Pre-speech and early speech development

Typical developmental patterns

The foundations for speech development occur in the first year of life with the emergence of vocalizations that serve as precursors for the production of words and phrases. Of particular importance to later speech development is the use of consonant-vowel syllables, such as [baba], which generally appear around 6 to 7 months (Oller, 1980). Phonetically, these 'canonical' babbles are similar, or even identical, to forms used in first words; thus, the phonetic form [mama] may be a non-meaningful babble at 8 months and a word at 14 months. The difference is awareness that words are based on an arbitrary relationship between sound and meaning. The timetable for development of babble and emergence of words is well documented, and is stable across socio-economic classes and different language environments. Hearing impairment, however, has been shown to cause substantial delays in the onset of canonical babble (Oller and Eilers, 1988; Stoel-Gammon and Otomo, 1986) and in the production of words.

In a typically developing child, first words appear around the end of the first year, overlapping with the period of late canonical babble; thereafter, babble and speech coexist for many months. When children have a productive vocabulary of about 10 different words, the proportion of words and babble in their spontaneous productions is roughly equal (Robb, Bauer and Tyler, 1994). When the productive vocabulary reaches 50 words, at around 18 months, the ratio of words to babble is about three to one.

During the transition to words, the phonetic characteristics of babble and speech are highly similar. Specifically, consonants that occur most frequently in babbling (stops, nasals, glides) also predominate in early word productions, while consonants that are infrequent in babble (fricatives, affricates, liquids) are precisely those that are acquired late in meaningful speech. Moreover, the consonant–vowel syllable structure, characteristic of canonical babbling period, is the most frequent syllabic type in early word productions. Thus, babbling and early speech share the same basic phonetic properties in terms of sound types and syllable structures (Stoel-Gammon, 1998).

There is a growing body of evidence linking pre-speech vocal development with general speech and language skills throughout early childhood (Stoel-Gammon, 1992). In general, increased use of complex babble in the prelinguistic period is linked to better performance on the speech and language measures after the onset of speech. Stoel-Gammon (1998) hypothesized that infants who produce more babble, particularly more canonical utterances with a variety of consonants and vowels, exhibit better early language skills because they have amassed a greater arsenal of 'building blocks' that can be recruited for the production of a wide variety of words.

Effects of Down syndrome

Although children with Down syndrome are delayed in the acquisition of speech and language skills, investigations of pre-speech development suggest that they are nearly typical in this domain. Dodd (1972) compared the babbling patterns of 10 infants with Down syndrome, and 10 typically developing infants. Despite differences on measures of mental and motor development, analyses of 15-minute recordings of spontaneous vocalizations revealed no significant differences between the two groups in terms of number of utterances, length of utterances, time spent vocalizing, and variety of consonant and vowel sounds produced. Dodd concluded that babbling does not reflect intelligence at this stage of development. Smith and Oller (1981) compared infants with Down syndrome with typically developing peers and reported similarities in age of onset of reduplicated canonical babble, place of articulation of consonants, and vowel quality. Longitudinal studies by Steffens, Oller, Lynch and Urbano (1992) and Smith and Stoel-Gammon (1996) also revealed that pre-speech patterns of infants with Down syndrome closely resemble those of typically developing peers.

In contrast to the studies cited above, Lynch and colleagues (Lynch, Oller, Steffens, Levine, Basinger, and Umbel, 1995) reported two differences in a longitudinal investigation of 13 infants with Down syndrome and 27 typically developing infants. First, the average age of onset of canonical babbling among the infants with Down syndrome was about 9 months, approximately two months later than the age for the typically developing infants. Second, over time, the occurrence of canonical babbling was less stable for the infants with Down syndrome. Hypotonicity and delays in motor development are characteristic of Down syndrome, so the relative instability in canonical babbling may be a consequence of deficits in the motor domain. These findings notwithstanding, it appears that Down syndrome has relatively little effect on pre-speech vocal development. In large measure, developmental patterns are within typical range, although the pre-speech period is much longer, often extending through the second year of life.

In contrast to the findings regarding pre-speech development, children with Down syndrome exhibit a substantial delay in the transition to meaningful speech and, once words appear, are slow to build an expressive vocabulary. Stray-Gunderson (1986) reported that some children produced words as early as 9 months (chronological age), within the range for children with typical development; for other children, first words did not appear until the age of 7. On average, however, word production was delayed. Buckley (2000) reported that the average productive vocabulary for 24-month-old children in her group with Down syndrome was 28 (compared with 250 for a typically developing child). At 3 years, the mean vocabulary was 116 words, rising to 248 words at 4 years, and to 330 words at 6 years, an age at which the child with typically development has a vocabulary of several thousand words. Other investigations of lexical acquisition in children with Down syndrome have shown that even when they are matched to a typically developing comparison group on mental (rather than chronological) age, lexical acquisition in children with Down syndrome is delayed (Chapman, 1997).

Single-word phonology

Typical developmental patterns

Phonological acquisition of children with typical development has been well documented. In the early stages, words are 'simplified' in terms of their structure: consonant clusters are reduced to single consonants, unstressed syllables are deleted, and consonants at the ends of words may be omitted. In terms of consonantal classes, stops, nasals and glides are generally acquired early, while fricatives, affricates and liquids are mastered later. Correct production of most vowels is achieved by 4 years (Stoel-Gammon and Herrington, 1990). Among children acquiring English, correct pronunciation of all phonemes is achieved by the age of 8 (Sander, 1972).

Effects of Down syndrome

A number of investigations of speech and language of individuals with mental retardation have reported that articulatory/phonological problems are particularly severe for children with Down syndrome (Blanchard 1968; Dodd 1975, 1976; Dodd and Leahy, 1989; Rosenberg and Abbeduto, 1993; Stoel-Gammon 1981). Production errors of these children resemble errors that occur in typical phonological development: fricatives, affricates and liquids have higher rates of error than stop, nasal and glide consonants (Bleile and Schwarz, 1984; Mackay and Hodson, 1982; Smith and Stoel-Gammon, 1983; Stoel-Gammon, 1981).

Analyses of error patterns (phonological processes) have also highlighted similarities between children with Down syndrome and those with typical development; in both groups, the following patterns are present:

* consonant clusters are produced as singleton consonants
* word-final consonants are omitted
* target fricatives and affricates are produced as stops
* aspirated voiceless stops in initial position are deaspirated
* word-initial liquids are produced as glides
* word-final liquids are produced as vowels or are omitted, and
* word-final voiced obstruents are devoiced (Bleiele and Schwarz, 1984; Cholmain, 1994; Dodd, 1976; Kumin, Councill and Goodman, 1994; Mackay and Hodson, 1982; Smith and Stoel-Gammon, 1983; Stoel-Gammon, 1980; Van Borsel, 1996).

Despite the similarities across groups, differences are also evident. Perhaps the most striking is rate of development. As might be expected, phonological development among children with Down syndrome proceeds at a slower rate than in their cognitively typical peers (Smith and Stoel-Gammon, 1983) and errors documented for young children with Down syndrome tend to persist through adolescence and into adulthood (Shriberg and Widder, 1990; Sommers, Reinhart and Sistrunk, 1988; Sommers, Patterson, and Wildgen, 1988).

In addition, the speech of children with Down syndrome exhibits more variability and a higher proportion of 'non-developmental' error types. Dodd (1976) compared the phonological systems of three groups of children matched for mental age: typical, intellectual disabled, and Down syndrome. The performance of children in the Down syndrome group differed from the other groups in several aspects. They made a greater number of phonological errors in their productions; their errors were more inconsistent; and a greater proportion of their errors could not be described by a set of common phonological processes. Stoel-Gammon (1981) also reported greater variability in errors, noting that children with typical development move from incorrect to correct phoneme production in a linear fashion with a small set of substitution types. In contrast, among children with Down syndrome, there was a greater range of substitution types and greater variation in errors from one word to another.

Intelligibility

Typical developmental patterns

Intelligibility (the degree to which speech can be understood) is influenced by a variety of causes, and the relationship between intelligibility and phonological skills is not straightforward. Initially, young children are often unintelligible to all but their immediate family. Between the ages of 2 and 4 years, intelligibility increases dramatically: At 2 years, approximately half (50%) of a child's productions can be understood by an adult not familiar with the child; at 3 years the proportion of intelligible productions rises to 75%; and at 4 years, it reaches 100% (Coplan and Gleason, 1988). Of course, this does not mean that a 4-year-old has acquired all the elements of the phonological system; rather, that the types of errors that remain have little impact on level of intelligibility.

Effects of Down syndrome

Unintelligibility is one of the characteristics associated with Down syndrome, and the speech of many individuals with Down syndrome tends to be unintelligible throughout their lives even though their mental age may exceed 4 years (Kumin 1994; Pueschel and Hopman, 1993; Shriberg and Widder, 1990). Long-standing difficulties with intelligibility can presumably be attributed to the array of speech production problems associated with Down syndrome.

Kumin (1994) surveyed 937 parents of children with Down syndrome aged birth to 40+ years; nearly 60% of the parents reported that, regardless of age, their child 'frequently' had difficulty being understood. An additional 37% reported that their children 'sometimes' had difficulty being understood. Pueschel and Hopman (1993) also used a questionnaire to gain information on parental views of their children's speech and language skills. Although these parents reported that their children, aged 4 to 21 years, were generally capable of making themselves understood, 71% to 94% noted that their offspring had problems with articulation.

Summary

Speech acquisition of children with Down syndrome follows a unique developmental path. Vocalizations in the first year of life are similar to those of infants with typical development in terms of onset of canonical babble and phonetic features of consonants and vowels produced. Whereas most children move from babble to meaningful speech toward the end of their first year, and acquire a productive vocabulary of 250 words by the age of 2 years, achievement of first words and development of an expressive vocabulary is considerably delayed in children with Down syndrome.

Phonological acquisition of children with Down syndrome follows typical patterns in terms of phoneme mastery and error types, although the rate of development is much slower. In addition, productions of the same word are often inconsistent, creating problems with speech intelligibility. Information from parents that intelligibility is a long-standing problem for individuals with Down syndrome.

Intervention strategies

Anatomical and structural differences

According to a number of authors, techniques for improving speech-motor deficits related to hypotonicity and possible hyposensitivity of the lip should be initiated in the first year of life. For example, Yarter (1980) suggests exercises that will strengthen the sucking response through use of a straw; lip stimulation; and encouraging the infant to 'mouth' objects. Kumin, Councill and Goodman (1994) suggest strengthening the orofacial musculature through a programme of lip massage, and bubble and whistle blowing for young children. They note that older children can be introduced to myofunctional exercises. While intervention techniques such as these are widely advocated for children with speech-motor delays, there is, to date, no evidence for claims that they enhance speech skills. Until such evidence is available, effects of these techniques are not known.

The most controversial approach to improving speech for children with Down syndrome is tongue reduction, a surgical procedure that is undertaken with the hope of increasing speech intelligibility, and diminishing problems with eating, breathing, and general appearance (Lemperle and Rodney, 1980; Olbrisch, 1982). Parsons, Iacono, and Rozner (1987) report the results of a study in which 18 children with Down syndrome underwent tongue-reduction surgery with the aim of increasing articulatory proficiency. The children's phonological skills were assessed preoperatively and postoperatively, and at a six-month follow-up. No significant differences in the number of articulation errors were found across this time period, and the articulation scores of the children undergoing the surgery were not significantly different than the scores of a non-surgery group. In spite of the lack of change in phonological skills, parents of the children in both the surgery and non-surgery groups claimed that their child's speech had improved during the period of the study.

Hearing

In terms of intervention related to hearing status, infants and children with Down syndrome should be treated for hearing loss associated with middle-ear pathology (Balkany, 1980; see also Downs, 1980). Recommendations include normalization of hearing through insertion of tympanostomy tubes and, in some cases, fitting of hearing aids; interruption of the cycle of recurrent otitis media with effusion through use of prophylactic drugs; and prevention of chronic ear disease through adequate otologic care. Yarter (1980) suggests that infants and young children should also receive an auditory training programme concurrently with their programme of speech therapy.

Pre-speech and early meaningful speech

The goal of intervention for infants/toddlers in the pre-speech period is to stimulate vocal productions and facilitate the transition to meaningful speech. Vocal stimulation focuses on increasing the frequency and diversity of speechlike babbles, with particular attention to production of canonical (consonant–vowel) syllables (Warren and Yoder, 1998). As noted in previous sections, use of canonical babble is correlated with subsequent speech and language development in infants with typical development (Stoel-Gammon, 1998) and those with developmental delays (McCathren, Yoder, and Warren, 1999). Thus, infants/toddlers whose pre-speech vocalizations include frequent consonant–vowel sequences productions and a relatively diverse phonetic repertoire can be expected to move more quickly to word productions and ultimately achieve better expressive language outcomes. Conversely, an extremely limited consonantal repertoire is likely to be associated with greater

delays in the acquisition of meaningful speech. For these children, some
have suggested that word training strategies be focused on the use of sign
rather than on speech (Wilcox and Shannon, 1998).

Facilitating the transition to speech is more complicated. As noted
earlier, in spite of relatively typical pre-speech skills, the onset of words is
significantly delayed in children with Down syndrome. Meaningful speech
productions require two elements: the ability to produce phonetic forms
that resemble words of the ambient language and the awareness that
sound production can be associated with meaning. Production of a form
like [ba] fulfils the phonetic aspect, and this is something many children
with Down syndrome can accomplish; linking a form like [ba] to a word
such as 'ball' or 'bottle' requires a representational link between sound
and meaning, and this is more difficult for children with Down syndrome.
One approach to increasing awareness of this relationship is to systematically link the child's vocalization of [ba] to the adult spoken form 'ball'
and to the object ball.

During the pre-speech period, intervention can take place at a special
setting (for example, a pre-school) with trained teachers or speech-language pathologists serving as agents (Warren, Yoder, Gazdag, Kim and
Jones, 1993). It can also take place in the home setting as the child interacts with parents or other caregivers. If parents are involved in the
intervention programme, it is important that they are aware of the goals,
so that they can provide the child with appropriate verbal models and
responses (Swift and Rosin, 1990).

Single-word phonology

Phonological intervention involves three steps:

* assessing the child's/client's phonological system
* setting the intervention goals, and
* determining the most appropriate methods for achieving those goals.

Phonological assessment for children with Down syndrome should
include information on phonetic inventory, syllables shapes, accuracy of
production, and nature of errors (see Le Prévost, Baksi, Pugh, and Clark,
2000 for a broad-based assessment protocol). In addition, consistency of
error types should be determined. Goal setting and decisions on type of
intervention are made on a case-by-case basis, with individual child factors
taken into account. For most children, a developmental model is adopted,
with syllable shapes and speech sounds that appear first in typical development targeted before later developing sounds and syllables shapes.

Most programmes focus on increasing the phonetic repertoire and
reducing the number of errors, using therapy techniques similar to those
for children with phonological delay or disorder. Cholmain (1994)
described a therapy programme for young children with Down syndrome

(chronological age 4;1–5;6) with unintelligible speech, and language ages between 1;4–2;10. The programme was designed to encourage the children to recognize the basic structures of the adult phonological system. Key elements of the programme included listening and production practice focused on particular phonemes and phonological processes, with therapy occurring in the clinic and at home. Results showed change in the children's phonological systems within the first two weeks of beginning therapy despite minimal change in the previous three to 12 months. Of particular interest is the fact that there were dramatic increases in the measure of percentage of consonants correct, with pre-therapy figures ranging from 3% to 38% and post-therapy figures (six to 14 weeks later) ranging from 19% to 88%. Marked improvements in the children's use of grammatical forms were also noted. The author concluded that the therapy approach allowed the children to restructure their sounds systems and proceed in syntax development.

Another type of therapy programme focused on the variability of word productions by Down-syndrome children (Dodd, McCormack and Woodyatt, 1994). This approach differs from traditional intervention programmes in two ways: the unit of treatment was whole words and parents served as the agents of therapy. Parents were instructed to accept only one pronunciation for a set of words individually selected for their child. Acceptable pronunciations could have errors as long as these were 'developmental' rather than 'deviant' errors. Over the 13-week programme, the four children in the study showed 'exceptional improvement' in the accuracy of production and the mean proportion of 'deviant' errors decreased substantially during the programme.

Intelligibility

Shriberg and Widder (1990) argue that in spite of the slow progress of children with Down syndrome and the limited resources of speech therapists and special education teachers, articulation therapy should remain as a high priority throughout childhood and adolescence. These authors note that improving the segmental and suprasegmental aspects of speech would increase intelligibility, which in turn would benefit social and vocational elements of individuals with mental handicap. In a similar vein, Fowler (1995) recommends to parents that they invest in speech therapy stating that it 'will provide your child with a greater sense of power to be understood' (p. 129).

Summary

In closing it should be remembered that speech therapy for children with Down syndrome takes different forms at different stages of development. Initially, the focus is on stimulating pre-speech vocalizations; then efforts are directed toward the use of speech in word productions; finally speech training involves efforts at improving the segmental and suprasegmental aspects of word, phrase and sentence productions with the goal of increasing levels of intelligibility. Speech therapy need not be the exclusive domain of therapists; parents, caregivers and educators can also be trained to serve as agents of therapy, thereby broadening the contexts in which therapy occurs and increasing the amount of intervention a child receives.

References

Balkany TJ (1980) Otologic aspects of Down's syndrome. Seminars in Speech, Language and Hearing 1: 39–48.

Blanchard I (1968) Speech pattern and etiology in mental retardation. American Journal of Mental Deficiency 68: 612–17.

Bleile K, Schwarz I (1984) Three perspectives on the speech of children with Down syndrome. Journal of Communication Disorders 17: 87–94.

Buckley SJ (2000) Speech and language development for individuals with Down syndrome – an overview. Portsmouth: The Down Syndrome Educational Trust.

Chapman RS (1997) Language development in children and adolescents with Down syndrome. Mental Retardation and Developmental Disabilities Research Reviews 3(4): 307–12.

Cholmain CN (1994) Working on phonology with young children with Down syndrome. Journal of Clinical Speech and Language Studies 1: 14–35.

Coplan J, Gleason J (1988) Unclear speech: recognition and significance of unintelligible speech in preschool children. Pediatrics 82: 447–52.

Dodd BJ (1972) Comparison of babbling patterns in normal and Down-syndrome infants. Journal of Mental Deficiency Research 16: 35–40.

Dodd BJ (1975) Recognition and reproduction of words by Down's syndrome and non-Down's syndrome retarded children. American Journal of Mental Deficiency 80: 306–11.

Dodd BJ (1976) A comparison of the phonological systems of mental age matched normal, severely abnormal and Down's syndrome children. British Journal of Disorders of Communication 11: 27–42.

Dodd BJ, Leahy P (1989) Phonological disorders and mental handicap. In M Beveridge, G Conti-Ramsden, I Leudar (eds) Language and Communication in Mentally Handicapped People. London: Chapman & Hall, pp. 33–56.

Dodd B, McCormack P, Woodyatt G (1994) Evaluation of an intervention program: Relation between children's phonology and parents' communicative behavior. American Journal of Mental Retardation 98(5): 632–45.

Downs MP (1980) The hearing of Down's individuals. Seminars in Speech, Language and Hearing 1: 25–37.

Fowler A (1995) Linguistic variability in persons with Down syndrome: research and implications. In L Nadel, D Rosenthal (eds) Down Syndrome: Living and Learning in the Community. New York: Wiley-Liss, pp. 121–31.

Kumin L (1994) Intelligibility of speech in children with Down syndrome in natural settings: parents' perspective. Perceptual and Motor Skills 78: 307–13.

Kumin L, Councill C, Goodman, M (1994) A longitudinal study of the emergence of phonemes in children with Down syndrome. Journal of Communication Disorders 27: 265–75.

Le Prévost P, Baksi L, Pugh D, Clark D (2000) Speech Intelligibility Profile for People with Down Syndrome. Unpublished manuscript.

Leddy M (1999) The biological bases of speech in people with Down syndrome. In JF Miller, M Leddy, LA Leavitt (eds) Improving the Communication of People with Down Syndrome. Baltimore: Paul H Brookes Co, pp. 61–80.

Lemperle G, Rodney D (1980) Facial plastic surgery in children with Down syndrome. Plastic and Reconstructive Surgery 66: 337–42.

Lynch MP, Oller DK, Steffens ML, Levine SL, Basinger DL, Umbel VM (1995) Development of speech-like vocalizations in infants with Down syndrome. American Journal of Mental Retardation 100: 68–86.

Mackay L, Hodson B (1982) Phonological process identification of misarticulations of mentally retarded children. Journal of Communication Disorders 15: 243–50.

McCathren RB, Yoder PJ, Warren SF (1999) The relationship between prelinguistic vocalization and later expressive vocabulary in young children with developmental delay. Journal of Speech, Language, and Hearing Research 42: 915–24.

Miller JF (1988) The developmental asynchrony of language development in children with Down syndrome. In L Nadel (ed.) The Psychobiology of Down Syndrome. Cambridge Mass: MIT Press, pp. 167–98.

Miller JF, Leddy M (1998) Down syndrome: the impact of speech production on language development. In R. Paul (ed.) Communication and Language Intervention Vol. 8. Exploring the Speech–Language Connection. Baltimore: Paul H. Brookes Publishing Co, pp. 163–77.

Olbrisch RR (1982) Plastic surgical management of children with Down's syndrome: implications and results. British Journal of Plastic Surgery 35: 195–200.

Oller DK (1980) The emergence of speech sounds in infancy. In GH Yeni-Komshian, CA Ferguson, J Kavanagh (eds) Child Phonology: Production. New York: Academic Press, vol. 1, pp. 93–112.

Oller DK, Eilers R (1988) The role of audition in infant babbling. Child Development 59: 441–9.

Parsons CL, Iacono TA, Rozner L (1987) Effect of tongue reduction on articulation in children with Down syndrome. American Journal of Mental Deficiency 91: 328–32.

Pueschel S, Hopman M (1993) Speech and language abilities of children with Down syndrome. In AP Kaiser, DB Gray (eds) Enhancing Children's Communication. Baltimore: Paul H Brookes, pp. 335–62.

Rast MM, Harris SR (1985) Motor control in infants with Down syndrome. Developmental Medicine and Child Neurology 27: 675–85.

Robb ML, Bauer HR, Tyler AA (1994) A quantitative analysis of the single word stage. First Language 14: 37–48.

Rosenberg S, Abbeduto L (1993) Language and Communication in Mental Retardation: Development, Process, and Intervention. Hillsdale NJ: Lawrence Erlbaum Associates.

Sander E (1972) When are speech sounds learned? Journal of Speech and Hearing Disorders 37: 55–63.

Shriberg L, Widder CJ (1990) Speech and prosody characteristics of adults with mental retardation. Journal of Speech and Hearing Research 33: 627–53.

Smith BL, Oller DK (1981) A comparative study of pre-meaningful vocalizations produced by normally developing and Down's syndrome infants. Journal of Speech and Hearing Disorders 46: 46–51.

Smith BL, Stoel-Gammon C (1983) A longitudinal study of the development of stop consonant production in normal and Down's syndrome children. Journal of Speech and Hearing Disorders 48: 114–18.

Smith BL, Stoel-Gammon C (1996) A quantitative analysis of the reduplicated and variegated babbling in vocalizations by Down syndrome infants. Clinical Linguistics and Phonetics 10: 119–30.

Sommers RK, Patterson JP, Wildgen PL (1988) Phonology of Down syndrome speakers, ages 13-22. Journal of Childhood Communication Disorders 12(1): 65–91.

Sommers RK, Reinhart RW, Sistrunk DA (1988) Traditional articulation measures of Down syndrome speakers, ages 13-22. Journal of Childhood Communication Disorders 12(1): 93–108.

Steffens ML, Oller DK, Lynch M, Urbano RC (1992) Vocal development in infants with Down syndrome and infants who are developing normally. American Journal of Mental Retardation 97: 235–46.

Stoel-Gammon C (1980) Phonological analysis of four Down's syndrome children. Applied Psycholinguistics 1: 31–48.

Stoel-Gammon C (1981) Speech development of infants and children with Down's syndrome. In JK Darby (ed.) Speech Evaluation in Medicine. New York: Grune & Stratton, pp. 341–60.

Stoel-Gammon C (1992) Prelinguistic vocal development: Measurement and predictions. In CA Ferguson, L Menn, C Stoel-Gammon (eds) Phonological Development: Models, Research, Implications. Timonium Md: York Press, pp. 439–56.

Stoel-Gammon C (1998) The role of babbling and phonology in early linguistic development. In AM Wetherby, SF Warren, J Reichle (eds) Transitions in Prelinguistic Communication: Preintentional to Intentional and Presymbolic to Symbolic. Baltimore: Paul H. Brookes Publishing Co, pp. 87–110.

Stoel-Gammon C, Herrington P (1990) Vowel systems of normally developing and phonologically disordered children. Clinical Linguistics and Phonetics 4: 145–60.

Stoel-Gammon C, Otomo K (1986) Babbling development of hearing-impaired and normally-hearing subjects. Journal of Speech and Hearing Disorders 51: 33–41.

Stray-Gunderson K (1986) Babies with Down syndrome: A New Parents Guide. Rockville Md: Woodbine House.

Swift E, Rosin P (1990) A remediation sequence to improve speech intelligibility for students with Down syndrome. Language, Speech, and Hearing Services in Schools 21: 140–6.

Van Borsel J (1996) Articulation in Down's syndrome adolescents and adults. European Journal of Disorders of Communication 31: 415–44.

Warren SF, Yoder PJ (1998) Facilitating the transition from preintentional to intentional communication. In AM Wetherby, SF Warren, J Reichle (eds) Communication and Language Intervention Vol. 7: Preintentional to Intentional and Presymbolic to Symbolic. Baltimore: Paul H. Brookes Publishing Co, pp. 365–84.

Warren SF, Yoder PJ, Gazdag GE, Kim K, Jones HA (1993) Facilitating prelinguistic communication skills in young children with developmental delay. Journal of Speech and Hearing Research 36: 83–97.

Wilcox MJ, Shannon MS (1998) Facilitating the transition from prelinguistic to linguistic communication. In AM Wetherby, SF Warren, J Reichle (eds) Transitions in Prelinguistic Communication: Preintentional to Intentional and Presymbolic to Symbolic. Baltimore: Paul H. Brookes Publishing Co, pp. 385–416.

Yarter BH (1980) Speech and language programs for the Down's population. Seminars in Speech, Language and Hearing 1: 49–61.

Chapter 5
Lexical development and intervention

CAROLYN B MERVIS, ANGELA M BECERRA

Words are the building blocks of language and verbal reasoning. Children begin to acquire concepts during the prelinguistic period; once language acquisition begins, words provide a means for children to communicate about these concepts to other people and to encode these concepts for themselves in an efficient manner. Words also serve to introduce children to new concepts. After children have acquired a critical mass of words (typically 50 to 100) in their productive vocabularies, they begin to produce word combinations. These combinations allow children to communicate efficiently about multiple concepts and about the relations among concepts. The ability to comprehend and produce words and word combinations provides the foundation not only for learning but also for peer relations. In this chapter, we briefly review the literature on acquisition of a basic vocabulary by young children with Down syndrome. We also consider the implications of this research for the design of interventions intended to facilitate the lexical development of children with Down syndrome.

Early words

We begin this section by reviewing studies of vocabulary size for young children with Down syndrome as a function of chronological age. These studies provide clear evidence that language acquisition for children with Down syndrome is delayed, and in many cases extremely delayed. Nevertheless, despite this quantitative difference in time of onset and rate of acquisition of new words, there are many similarities in the progression of early lexical development for children with Down syndrome and typically developing children. These similarities (as well as some differences) are discussed in the remainder of this section. First, relations between early lexical and sensorimotor development, early lexical comprehension and gestural development, early lexical comprehension and production, and early lexical production and grammatical development are considered. Second, similarities in the content of the early vocabularies of children with Down syndrome and typically developing children are discussed. Finally, similarities in the initial extension patterns of the early object words of children with Down syndrome and typically developing children and in the evolution of these patterns to conform to the adult extensions are addressed.

Quantitative measures of vocabulary size

Until recently, it was very difficult to determine the size of young children's vocabularies. Recordings of parent-child interactions (for example, play sessions) consistently lead to underestimates of vocabulary size for at least two reasons. First, young children talk less when they are in new settings or around people they do not know. Second, it is impossible during a play session to simulate the wide variety of situations in which a child produces language, and much of the language that a young child produces is relatively situation-specific. Asking parents to recall all the words they have heard their child produce also is likely to result in an underestimate because of the demands associated with recall from long-term memory. A much better method is to provide parents with a list of words and ask them to indicate which of the words they have heard their child produce spontaneously (not in imitation of someone else). Parents also can be asked to indicate which words their child understands, even though he or she does not yet produce them. The checklist method relies on recognition memory rather than recall. There is now a normed 680-word checklist for English, the MacArthur Communicative Development Inventory: Words and Sentences (CDI; Fenson et al., 1993), which has been shown to have high validity both for typically developing children (Fenson et al., 1994) and children who have Down syndrome (Miller, Sedey and Miolo, 1995). Similar checklists have been developed or are being developed for a variety of other languages. The availability of these checklists has permitted a much better understanding of children's vocabulary sizes as a function of chronological age.

Typically developing children usually produce their first words by about age 12 months. For the next six months or so they add new words to their productive vocabulary at a slow but gradually increasing rate, resulting in a median productive vocabulary size of about 70 words at age 17 months (Fenson et al., 1993; fifth percentile to 95th percentile: ~15 to ~260 words). At this point most typically developing children evidence a vocabulary spurt at the peak of which some children add as many as 40 or 50 new words to their productive vocabulary in a single week. By age 24 months, the median vocabulary size for typically developing children is about 320 words (Fenson et al., 1993; fifth percentile to 95th percentile:

~60 to ~640 words). Shortly after the vocabulary spurt begins, most typically developing children begin to produce two-word combinations.

The onset of productive language for children who have Down syndrome is almost always delayed. Berglund, Eriksson and Johansson (2001) in a study of 330 Swedish children with Down syndrome, found that only 12% of their sample of 1-year-olds (age range 1;0 to 1;11) produced any words; only 3% produced 10 or more words. Of their 2-year-old sample (age range 2;0 to 2;11), 80% produced at least one word, 53% produced 10 or more words, and 3% produced 50 or more words. The 4-year-old sample (age range 4;0 to 4;11) was the youngest one in which half of the children (53%) had productive vocabularies of at least 50 words. This is about the median vocabulary size for a typically developing 16-month-old (Fenson et al., 1993). In Berglund et al.'s study, only spoken words were included in the child's productive vocabulary; signs were excluded. The authors state that this procedure slightly underestimates the total productive vocabulary of the younger children in the sample.

Six additional studies of the vocabulary sizes of toddlers and preschoolers with Down syndrome using the CDI have been published: four of children acquiring English and two of children acquiring Italian. In each of these studies, a word was considered to be part of the child's productive lexicon if the child either said or signed the word spontaneously (not in imitation of another speaker). The findings from these studies are summarized in Table 5.1. Berglund et al. (2001) is not included in the table because mean vocabulary sizes were not reported for the different age groups. All six studies confirm that the extensive delay in expressive vocabulary development that Berglund et al. (2001) reported for children with Down syndrome learning Swedish as a native language, is also characteristic of children with Down syndrome learning English or Italian as their native language. Results for individual children relative to CDI norms were presented in only one paper. Mervis and Robinson (2000) reported that of the 13 children in their sample who were young enough (2;6 or less) for the CDI norms to be applicable, 12 had productive vocabularies below the 5th percentile (the lowest percentile included in the CDI norms); the remaining child's productive vocabulary size was at the 8th percentile.

The question of whether children with Down syndrome evidence a vocabulary spurt has been addressed in several studies. Based on cross-sectional data, Berglund et al. (2001) concluded that vocabulary growth for children with Down syndrome as a group was best fit by a logistic or exponential function, suggesting that most children with Down syndrome eventually do evidence a vocabulary spurt. Miller (1992, 1999), using cross-sectional data derived from an earlier version of the CDI and measuring age by mental age rather than chronological age, also found that children with Down syndrome as a group evidence a vocabulary spurt, but that this spurt occurs at a considerably older mental age than for typically developing children. Oliver and Buckley (1994), using longitudinal diaries of vocabulary acquisition kept by parents of young children with Down syndrome, found that some, but not all, of the children evidenced a vocabulary spurt during the course of the study. Mervis, Robinson, and Bertrand (1998), using the CDI, found that about half of the children with Down syndrome in their longitudinal sample showed logistic vocabulary growth, clear evidence that they had had a vocabulary spurt during the course of the study. It is likely that many of the children who had not had a vocabulary spurt prior to the end of the studies in which they participated, did have a spurt later.

Table 5.1. Expressive vocabulary size as measured by the Communicative Development Inventories, as a function of chronological age.

Authors	Language	N	Chronological age		Productive vocabulary size		
			Mean	Range	Mean	S.D.	Range
Caselli et al. (1998)	Italian	40	2;5	0;10 – 4;1	27	55.5	0 – 302
Kumin et al. (1998, 1999)	English	27	n.a.	2;0 – 2;11	55	n.a.	8 – 226
Mervis & Robinson (2000)	English	28	2;6	2;0 – 2;11	66	79.24	0 – 324
Miller et al. (1995)	English	20	2;10	2;5 – 3;6	42	38.71	2 – 144
Kumin et al. (1998, 1999)	English	31	n.a.	3;0 – 3;11	168	n.a.	5 – 675
Miller et al. (1995)	English	20	3;10	3;5 – 4;7	168	134.48	9 – 440
Singer Harris et al. (1997)	English	23	3;11	2;6 – 5;8	252	195.0	n.a.
Kumin et al. (1998, 1999)	English	34	n.a.	4;0 – 4;11	251	n.a.	22 – 675
Kumin et al. (1998, 1999)	English	23	n.a.	5;0 – 5;11	391	n.a.	62 – 611
Vicari et al. (2000)	Italian	15	5;5	4;0 – 6;2	420	159.2	n.a.

Relations between early lexical acquisition and other aspects of development

Early lexical acquisition and sensorimotor development

The relation between early language acquisition and Piagetian stages of sensorimotor development for object permanence and means–ends relations has been addressed in several studies of typically developing children (for example, Corrigan, 1978; Folger and Leonard, 1978). Findings indicate that typically developing children usually begin to comprehend referential language during stage five of object permanence development and produce referential language during stage six. For means–ends relations, referential comprehension begins during stage five (functional use of objects); most children are still in stage five at the start of referential production of language. The onset of referential comprehension or production in stage four of either object permanence or means–ends relations was extremely rare.

The relations between these aspects of sensorimotor development and language acquisition have been considered in only one study of children with Down syndrome. Cardoso-Martins, Mervis and Mervis (1985) studied the early language development of six children with Down syndrome and six typically developing children longitudinally, from before the onset of referential comprehension. Both the children with Down syndrome and the typically developing children showed the same patterns of relations between sensorimotor development and early language acquisition as were found in earlier studies of typically developing children. At the onset of referential comprehension, three of the children with Down syndrome and four of the typically developing children were in stage five of object permanence development; the remaining children were in stage six. At the onset of referential production, all of the children in both groups were in stage six of object permanence; at this time, five of the children in each group were in stage five of means–ends relations, with the remaining children in stage six.

Although the onset of referential comprehension and referential production in the Cardoso-Martins et al. (1985) study occurred at the same sensorimotor level for children with Down syndrome and typically developing children, rate of vocabulary acquisition for the two groups relative to rate of sensorimotor development was quite different. Children with Down syndrome had significantly smaller comprehension vocabulary sizes than typically developing children both at the time of complete attainment of stage five of object permanence and at the time of complete attainment of stage six. Comprehension vocabulary size was also significantly smaller for the children with Down syndrome at the time of complete attainment of stage five of means–ends relations. The children with Down syndrome had significantly smaller productive vocabulary sizes than the typically developing children at complete attainment of stage six of object permanence. Too few children with Down syndrome completed stage six of means–ends relations during the study to justify analyses of vocabulary size at this attainment.

Early lexical acquisition and early gestural development

Referential pointing gestures are used by both children and adults to draw others' attention to interesting objects or events, producing joint attention to the same referent. In this situation, adults often label the referent of the pointing gesture, providing a particularly supportive framework for children acquiring their first words (Masur, 1982). Thus, comprehension and production of referential pointing gestures should facilitate the child's lexical acquisition. Typically developing children usually comprehend and produce referential pointing gestures prior to producing referential language (for example, Carpenter, Nagell and Tomasello, 1998). The same pattern has been shown for children with Down syndrome (Greenwald and Leonard, 1979; Smith, Von Techner, and Michalsen, 1988). Franco and Wishart (1995) found that when matched for language age, children with Down syndrome produced significantly more referential pointing gestures than typically developing children did, both during the prelinguistic period and during the early period of lexical acquisition. Thus, a solid gestural foundation for language is well established for children with Down syndrome at the time they begin to acquire language.

The Words and Gestures version of the CDI (Fenson et al., 1993) includes parental report of children's early gestures, using a checklist format. Both communicative gestures (for example, pointing, reaching) and functional, symbolic play, and pretending gestures (for example, pushing a toy car, feeding a bottle to a stuffed animal, 'playing' an instrument) are included. Norms are available comparing children's level of gesturing ability (collapsed across all types of gestures) to their expressive and receptive vocabulary sizes. Singer Harris et al. (1997) found that children with Down syndrome showed more advanced gesturing ability than expected based on both their receptive and expressive vocabulary sizes (79th and 81st percentiles, respectively). Of the 28 participants with Down syndrome, 25 were above the 50th percentile on these measures. Caselli et al. (1998), using the Italian version of the CDI: Words and Gestures, also found a gestural advantage for children with Down syndrome, beginning at the 100-word receptive vocabulary level. This advantage was primarily for functional, symbolic play, and pretending gestures – gestures that involve more advanced cognitive skills. Combined, the results of the Franco and Wishart (1995) study and the two CDI studies suggest that children with Down syndrome both produce more referential pointing gestures and have a wider repertoire of functional, symbolic and pretending gestures than do typically developing children at the same language level.

At the same time, young children with Down syndrome are significantly less likely to produce imperative (requesting) pointing gestures than typically developing children matched for language age (Sigman and Ruskin, 1999). This reduced use of imperative gestures relative to typically developing children is not unique to children with Down syndrome; Sigman and Ruskin found the same pattern for children with autism and children with developmental delays of mixed etiology.

Early lexical comprehension and production

Receptive vocabulary size is expected to be larger than expressive vocabulary size for all children, whether they have a disability or not. However, it is possible to determine if the relation between productive vocabulary size and receptive vocabulary size for children with Down syndrome (or any other disability) is similar to that for typically developing children, using norms from the CDI: Words and Gestures. This comparison has been made for children with Down syndrome in two studies. In both studies, productive vocabulary size was found to be at the level expected for receptive vocabulary size. Singer Harris et al. (1997) found that, for the children with Down syndrome in their sample, the mean percentile for productive vocabulary size relative to receptive vocabulary size was 60. Caselli et al. (1998) reported that there was no difference between the children with Down syndrome and the typically developing children in their sample for this measure. Thus, during the early period of lexical acquisition, the relation between expressive and receptive vocabulary size is the same as that found for typically developing children.

Early lexical production and grammatical development

On average, typically developing children begin to combine words when their productive vocabulary size reaches 50 to 100 words. Children with Down syndrome also begin to combine words at this time. Oliver and Buckley (1994) reported a mean vocabulary size of 54 words (range: 21 to 109) at the time their sample of children with Down syndrome first produced two-word phrases. Berglund et al. (2001) found that for each of the vocabulary sizes that they considered, children with Down syndrome were as likely as typically developing children to have begun to combine words. Berglund also found that the order of grammatical development for children with Down syndrome acquiring Swedish as a native language was the same as for typically developing children: First, children began to combine words; then they produced possessive markers followed by use of definite singulars and plurals and indefinite singulars and plurals; use of past tense markers was last.

However, although the onset of word combinations and the order of acquisition of grammatical markers are similar for children with Down syndrome and typically developing children, the rate at which grammatical development proceeds relative to rate of productive vocabulary growth differs. Based on norms for the CDI: Words and Sentences, Singer Harris et al. (1997) found a mean percentile of 32 for grammatical complexity relative to productive vocabulary size for children with Down syndrome. Eleven of the 14 children with Down syndrome in this sample were below the 50th percentile. Berglund et al. (2001) reported that for comparable vocabulary sizes, children with Down syndrome were less likely than typically developing children to use possessive, indefinite singular, and definite singular markers. Vicari, Caselli and Tonucci (2000) compared a group of children with Down syndrome with a group of younger typically developing children matched for productive vocabulary size (means of ~450 words) on the Italian version of the CDI: Words and Sentences. Results for the Sentence Complexity scale of the CDI indicated that the children with Down syndrome on average used simpler, more telegraphic sentences than the typically developing children. Mean length of utterance, based on a spontaneous language sample, was also significantly lower for the children with Down syndrome than for the typically developing children. Moreover, the children with Down syndrome made many more errors than the typically developing children when asked to repeat a sentence presented in the context of a picture illustrating the sentence. Increased error rates were reported for all word types: articles, nouns, verbs, modifiers, and prepositions. However, the relative error rates for the different word types were similar for the two groups of children.

Early vocabulary: content

The early words produced by young children are not a random subset of the words that they hear. This is not surprising; at the start of lexical acquisition, both comprehension and production are quite difficult for the young child. Thus, children are likely to learn names only for people, objects, or activities in which they have great interest (Mervis, 1983). Nelson (1973, p. 33) noted that the first words of typically developing children refer primarily to people or objects that have 'salient properties of change', that is, entities that either can move independently or can be manipulated by the child. Bloom (2000) has argued that at the start of language acquisition, words are learned only for items or activities that are not only salient but are also of emotional interest to the child, providing him or her with sufficient motivation to learn their labels. These characteristics are true of the first words of children with Down syndrome as well. Oliver and Buckley (1994) studied nine children longitudinally from the beginning of lexical production. The most common first words were 'daddy', 'mommy', 'bye-bye', and a person's name. The most common early words for typically developing children (based on the CDI frequency norms reported in Dale and Fenson, 1996) were also 'daddy', 'mommy', and 'bye-bye'. More generally, the first 10 words produced both by children with Down syndrome and typically developing children are primarily names for people, labels for whole objects (for example, kitty, ball), or words referring to routines (bye-bye, uh-oh); labels for object parts, action words, and descriptive words are very rare (Gillham, 1979; Mervis, 1983, 1990; Oliver and Buckley, 1994).

Any object can be categorized and labelled at multiple hierarchical levels. Psychologists and educators usually consider three levels: subordinate (for example, collie, Macintosh apple), basic (for example, dog, apple), and superordinate (for example, animal, fruit). Rosch, Mervis, Gray, Johnson, and Boyes-Braem (1976) argued that the basic level is the most salient psychologically. This is the most general level at which category members have similar overall shapes (formed of clusters of correlated attributes) and similar characteristic action patterns or functions (based on the correlated form attributes). Consequently, children would be expected to learn labels at this level first, and parents would be expected to label objects for their children primarily at this level. The results of an examination of the language diary records for 47 typically developing children confirm that these children learned to label objects at the basic level before learning their superordinate or subordinate names (Mervis, 1983). Studies of children with Down syndrome also confirm the priority of basic-level labels over labels at other hierarchical levels

(Gillham, 1979; Mervis, 1990; Mervis and Bertrand, 1997; Oliver and Buckley, 1994). Mervis (1990) reported that although the children with Down syndrome in her longitudinal study comprehended the basic level names for the toys used in the play sessions by age 36 months, very few of the children comprehended the subordinate names for any of these toys, and none of the children produced any subordinate labels for them. Mervis and Bertrand (1997), using a checklist format completed by parents, also found that children with Down syndrome almost always comprehended the basic level name of an object before comprehending its subordinate level name. As expected, based on the literature for typically developing children (see summary in Mervis, 1983), parents of children with Down syndrome primarily labelled objects with their basic level name, and when subordinate names were introduced, it was usually in the context of the object's basic level name (for example, 'this kind of dog is called a collie').

Early object words: initial extension

The most basic category formation principle is the form–function principle: the form and function of objects are noticeably correlated; use this correlation as the basis for categorization (Mervis, 1990; Mervis, Mervis, Johnson, and Bertrand, 1992). By the age of 10 months, typically developing children are able to apply this principle to form categories (Mervis, Pani, and Pani, in press). Children with Down syndrome are not able to use this principle at age 10 months. However, they are able to use it prior to beginning to comprehend language referentially (Mervis, 1987; Mervis and Bertrand, 1997).

The form–function principle provides the foundation for categorization and therefore for naming for both children and adults. Nevertheless, young children's early categories are usually not identical to those labelled by adults with the same name. These differences occur because very young children and adults may attend to different attributes of the same object, as a function of different experiences or different levels of expertise (Mervis, 1987). Very young children often do not share adults' knowledge of culturally appropriate functions of particular objects and the form attributes correlated with those functions, so these children may de-emphasize attributes that are important from an adult perspective. At the same time, very young children may notice a function (and its correlated form attributes) for that object that adults ignore, leading the children to emphasize features that are unimportant to adults. In these situations, child-basic categories will differ systematically from the corresponding adult-basic categories. For example, results of research with both typically developing children and children with Down syndrome indicate that the child-basic *ball* category typically includes not only baseballs, basketballs, and tennis balls, but also spherical candles, spherical coin banks, and spherical or multisided beads – objects that adults would not consider to be balls, but that nevertheless are ball shaped and can roll. At the same time, very young children may exclude American-type or rugby footballs from their *ball* category because an American football's overall shape is not spherical and does not roll in the same manner as typical balls (Mervis, 1984, 1987; Mervis and Bertrand, 1997).

When young children's categories do not correspond exactly to the adult categories labelled by the same name, children's categories may be overextended, underextended, or may overlap the adult category. Overextended categories include all the objects that adults would include, as well as additional ones. Underextended categories exclude some of the objects that adults would include, but do not include any additional objects. Overlapped categories include some but not all of the objects adults would include, and at the same time include some objects that adults would exclude. When very young children are carefully tested, the most common relation that emerges between child-basic level categories and the adult-basic level categories labelled by the same name, is overlap. This relation holds for both typically developing children and children with Down syndrome (Mervis, 1984, 1987, 1990).

Interestingly, at the time that children first begin to acquire object labels, children sometimes do not assign objects to the categories corresponding to the labels provided by adults for those objects. Instead, labels are extended based on the child's prelinguistic categories. Mothers of typically developing children often label objects to correspond with the categories to which they expect their child to assign an object. Thus, these mothers are likely to label spherical banks, 'ball' and leopards, 'kitty.' However, mothers of children with Down syndrome typically label objects with their correct (from an adult perspective) basic level name and sometimes try to prevent the child from using an object in a child-basic manner (for example, rolling a spherical candle). Despite these differences in input, however, both typically developing children and children with Down syndrome form the same initial child-basic categories (as measured by lexical comprehension and production), including objects that the child considers to fit the form–function correlation underlying the category (for example leopards and tigers in the *kitty* category) and excluding objects that the child considers not to fit this correlation (for example, flat, flowered cotton housecat-shaped sachets, live hairless housecats), regardless of how these are labelled by their communicative partners (Mervis, 1984, 1987).

Early object words: evolution of initial extension to correspond to adult extension

Children's initial child-basic categories and category labels eventually evolve to correspond to the adult-basic categories and category labels. A critical component in this evolution is the provision of the adult-basic category label by the child's communicative partner, for an object that the child has not included in that category. There are four different types of circumstances under which adults provide 'correct' labels for objects that the child considers to be members of a different category, thus providing the child with an opportunity to learn the 'correct' label and to change his or her categorization scheme accordingly. First, the child might notice attributes of the object important to its adult category assignment and call these attributes to the adult's attention. For example, one of the children in Mervis's (1983) study bit into a spherical candle, made a face, and then held the candle out to her mother, saying, 'yucky ball'. Her mother responded by saying 'that's a candle!' Later that afternoon, the child demonstrated comprehension of the word 'candle' in reference to spherical candles. If the child does not point these attributes out to the adult, the adult could point them out to the child at the same time as providing the adult-basic label. The adult could provide both a verbal description of one or more important form or function attributes and a concrete demonstration of the attribute (for example, for a spherical bank, the adult could show the child the slot, insert a coin, and then tell the child that this is a special hole you put money in) at the same time as labelling the object, 'bank'. Alternatively, the adult could provide a verbal description without a demonstration. Finally, the adult could label the object with its adult-basic name without either an implicit request from the child (the first circumstance described) or some form of explanation (the second and third circumstances).

The four circumstances are differentially associated with success in inducing the child to comprehend the adult-basic label for an object for which he or she already has a child-basic label, allowing the process of category evolution to begin. Results from longitudinal studies both of typically developing children and children with Down syndrome (such as Mervis, 1990; Mervis et al., in press) indicate that early in the language acquisition process, the first two circumstances are most likely to lead to the child's comprehension of the new label. Although during this period children (especially children with disabilities, including Down syndrome) quite often hear the object labelled with its adult-basic name without any explanation (the fourth circumstance), they only rarely learn the new label based on this type of input. For example, Mervis (1990) found that during the course of her longitudinal study (through age 36 to 39 months) only the first two strategies were successful in inducing children with Down syndrome to comprehend the adult-basic category name for an object already included in a different child-basic category. As children acquire more language, attribute descriptions without demonstrations (the third strategy) become more likely to succeed. Eventually, once children realize that adults are the most likely ones to know the correct names for objects (the expert principle), new labels will be acquired and category evolution begun based on adult provision of the correct name without any additional information (fourth strategy).

Comprehension of the adult-basic name for an object already included in a child-basic category with a different label is the first step in the evolution of that category to conform to the adult-basic category labelled by the same word. For very young children, whether typically developing or with Down syndrome or other forms of developmental delay, the complete separation of the old and new categories usually is gradual, occurring only when the child decides that only the set of attributes that makes the object a member of the new category is important (Mervis, 1987, 1990; Mervis et al., in press). Once children have acquired the expert principle, immediate separation of the old and new categories becomes the norm (Mervis et al., in press).

Lexical development beyond first words

Most of the research on lexical development of children with Down syndrome has focused on the earliest stages of this process. A few studies of the next stages of lexical development have been conducted, however, focusing on fast mapping of novel object names and on the acquisition of internal state vocabulary.

Fast mapping of novel object names

During the early stages of lexical development, children typically learn object names only if the referent is made clear to them, for example because the speaker or child is pointing to the object or the child was already attending to the object. Usually the object needs to be named multiple times before the child comprehends it. At about 18 months, however, most typically developing children begin to be able to acquire new object labels even when the adult does not make the referent so explicit or does not label the referent multiple times (Mervis and Bertrand, 1994; Tomasello, 2001). For example, the child realizes that when a speaker produces a new label in the context of a variety of objects including one for which the child does not yet have a name, the new label is probably the name for that object, the 'novel name – novel category (N3C) principle' (Mervis and Bertrand, 1994, 1995). This process is referred to as fast mapping (e.g., Carey, 1978).

Chapman, Kay-Raining Bird and Schwartz (1990) conducted the first study of fast mapping by individuals with Down syndrome. In this study, conducted as a hiding game, participants were shown four objects, two familiar and two unfamiliar, and were asked to hide the named object in a particular location. After the child had hidden the two familiar objects and one of the unfamiliar objects, the experimenter told him or her where to hide the 'koob'. No gestural support (such as pointing) was provided. All of the participants responded by hiding the correct object. The experimenter then retrieved the four objects, arranged them plus an additional unknown object in a line and asked the child first to give her one of the known objects and then to give her the 'koob'. Of the youngest group of children with Down syndrome (ages 5;6 – 8;5), 62% responded correctly to the request for the 'koob', a rate equivalent to that of mental age-matched typically developing children. Generalization of the new label to another member of the 'koob' category was not tested.

Mervis and Bertrand (1995) considered the fast mapping abilities of younger children with Down syndrome (ages 2;5 – 3;4), using a procedure similar to that of Carey's (1978) original fast-mapping study. Children were shown four sets of five objects (four with names the child knew and one whose name the child did not know) and asked to give the experimenter one of the known objects and the unknown object, which was labelled with a nonsense word. Order of testing for the known and unknown objects was counterbalanced. After the child had been tested on two sets of objects, he or she was tested for generalization of the new labels to additional members of the unknown category; in these trials, two unknown objects were included (an additional member of the category labelled by the nonsense word and an object that was clearly not a member of the labelled category) as well as three familiar objects. The procedure was the same as for the original trials. Finally, the child's comprehension of the new labels was tested the next day using the same procedure. Results indicated that about half of the children were able to fast map new object labels. These children also were able to generalize the new labels to other members of the category and were able to comprehend the category labels the next day. The children who were able to fast map did not differ in age from the children who could not fast map. However, the fast mappers had significantly larger comprehension and production vocabulary sizes as measured by the CDI, and their mothers spontaneously reported that they had been acquiring new words at a rapid rate. None of the parents of the children who were unable to fast map reported that their child's vocabulary was growing rapidly. These results confirm that fast mapping is a relatively late developing ability that is related to a substantially increased rate of vocabulary acquisition.

Acquisition of internal state vocabulary

Internal state words refer to sensory perception, physiology, positive and negative affect, affective behaviour, moral judgement, obligation, volition, and cognition. These words reflect children's emerging self-awareness and differentiation of themselves from others; this knowledge is often considered to underlie the regulation of social interaction (Dunn and Brown, 1991). Although some internal state words may be acquired relatively early (for example, 'see', 'want', 'kiss', 'sleepy', 'hot'), most are acquired after children have amassed a basic vocabulary of object, action, and routine words. By age 30–36 months, typically developing children have a solid vocabulary of internal state words, although these words do not yet have their full adult meaning (Beeghly and Cicchetti, 1997). The development of internal state language by children with Down syndrome has been examined in only one study. Beeghly and Cicchetti (1997) compared the internal state language of two groups of children with Down syndrome to mental age-matched typically developing children. The younger group of children with Down syndrome had a mean chronological age of 3;6 and a mean mental age of 1;10; the older group had a mean chronological age of 6;5 and a mean mental age of 3;10. Internal state language was derived from two sources: mother–child conversation while looking at a picture book composed of photographs of children in a variety of emotionally charged situations and a mother–children free play session with a set of toys chosen by the experimenter. Results indicated substantial growth in internal state language by children with Down syndrome; the older group used a significantly more varied internal state vocabulary than the younger group (means of 2.8 and 9.0 different words, respectively). Furthermore, whereas more than half of the internal state words used by the younger group referred to perception, the internal state vocabulary of the older group was more varied, including a substantially larger proportion of moral judgement/obligation and ability words. Older children with Down syndrome also were more likely to use internal state words in a decontextualized manner than were younger children. Finally, use of internal state words was strongly correlated with MLU; children with more advanced grammatical development also had more varied internal state vocabulary and were more likely to use these words in a decontextualized manner. These developmental patterns were shown by the typically developing children as well. However, despite being matched for mental age, the typically developing children were considerably more advanced than the children with Down syndrome with regard to the size of their internal state vocabulary, their ability to use it in a decontextualized manner, and proportional use of more abstract types of internal state words. These differences were especially pronounced for the older groups.

Factors that influence lexical development

Rate of lexical development is influenced by both the quantity and quality of joint attention episodes between children and adults, as well as by the child's auditory memory abilities. Each of these factors is considered briefly.

Joint attention

In order for children to determine the referent of a word, they must be attending to the same object or action as the speaker. This joint attention can occur either because the adult follows in to the child's focus of attention or because the adult redirects the child's attention. Tomasello and Farrar (1986) found that at age 15 months, four types of maternal joint object reference were positively associated with vocabulary size for typically developing children. Three types involved the mother following in to the child's focus of attention and then labelling it. The fourth type involved the mother redirecting the child's focus of attention by gesturing (e.g., pointing) to a different object and then providing its name. However, by age 21 months, the redirecting method was significantly negatively correlated with vocabulary size; greater use of this method was associated with smaller vocabulary sizes. In contrast, the following-in methods continued to provide solid support for vocabulary acquisition, as indicated by significant positive correlations with vocabulary size.

Harris, Kasari and Sigman (1996) have examined the impact of joint attention on language acquisition of young children with Down syndrome. Joint attention was measured during a mother–child play period during the first session of the study. Language level was measured at both sessions. At the time of the first visit, the mean chronological age for the children with Down syndrome was 1;11 and the mean mental age was 1;5. At the second visit, mean chronological age was 3;0 and mean mental age was 2;0. A comparison group of typically developing children matched for mental age at the first visit was also included. Results indicated that the two groups of mothers were equally likely to maintain joint attention to toys selected by their child, and both groups were equally likely to redirect their child. However, mothers of children with Down syndrome were significantly more likely than mothers of typically developing children to maintain attention to adult-selected toys. Correlations between joint attention measures derived from the first visit and amount of language gain between the two visits indicate that for both typically developing children and children with Down syndrome, maternal maintenance of attention to child-selected topics was significantly positively correlated with child receptive language gain. For both groups of children, there was also a significant negative correlation between maternal redirection of child attention and child receptive language gain.

Verbal memory

Phonological, or verbal working, memory ability is strongly related to vocabulary size for typically developing children (Baddeley, Gathercole and Papagno, 1998). In Conners' review of the literature on the verbal memory abilities of children with Down syndrome (this volume; see also Jarrold, Baddeley and Phillips, 1999), she reported that children with Down syndrome consistently evidence difficulty with verbal short-term memory. The difficulty has been localized to the phonological store component of memory. Thus, it is not surprising that children and adults with Down syndrome have smaller vocabularies than expected for their chronological age. Both Conners (this volume) and Jarrold et al. (1999) argue that the memory difficulty evidenced by individuals with Down syndrome is localized to the phonological loop component of verbal working memory, more specifically to the phonological store.

Two case studies of young adults with Down syndrome who have good verbal memory abilities have been reported (Vallar and Papagno, 1993; Rondal, 1995). Both of these individuals had phonological memory abilities that were near the mean of the general population. Backward digit span (a measure of verbal working memory) reported for only one of the cases was also within one standard deviation of the mean for the general population. In contrast, control individuals with Down syndrome had markedly shorter forward digit spans, nonsense word repetition spans (a measure of phonological working memory), and backward digit spans. Both of the individuals with Down syndrome who had good verbal memory also had good vocabulary ability; scaled scores for the vocabulary subtest of the WAIS were within one standard deviation of the mean for the general population. In contrast, the vocabulary abilities of the control adults with Down syndrome were well below the normal range. These case studies provide further support for the importance of verbal short-term memory abilities for vocabulary acquisition.

Lexical intervention

Mervis (1990) stated that intervention concerned with early vocabulary acquisition should have three interrelated goals. First, the child and the adults who interact with him or her should develop patterns of interaction that are comfortable and effective for all of them. Second, the child should learn, and learn correctly (initially from the child perspective and eventually from the adult perspective) as many words as possible. Third, the child should be encouraged to use the words he or she knows spontaneously, both to express ideas and to attempt to control the environment. In this section, we offer suggestions for how to implement these goals, based on prior research.

Establishing a comfortable and effective environment: the importance of joint attention and wait time

Virtually every article on language intervention published in the past two decades has stressed the importance of establishing and maintaining joint attention for facilitating children's lexical development (for example, Girolametto, Weitzman, and Clements-Baartman, 1998; Kaiser, Hester, and McDuffie, 2001). It is common sense that it would be extremely difficult for a child to learn new words if he or she is not attending to the object or event the speaker has labelled. As we reviewed earlier in this chapter, research has established that the most effective form of joint attention involves the adult following in on the focus of the child's attention and then labelling that focus. Maintaining the child's attention to that object or event and labelling it multiple times within the same episode, as well as across different episodes, is especially important for young children who are just beginning to acquire language. This approach is particularly important for young children with Down syndrome, whose verbal memory weaknesses greatly increase the difficulty of encoding and remembering new words and their referents. It is greatly preferable for the adult to follow in on the child's focus of attention rather than attempting to switch the child's focus; switching focus requires cognitive resources that the child otherwise could allocate to attending to the adult language. Furthermore, when children first begin to talk, they learn labels only for objects or events that are particularly motivating to them; in most cases, these will be objects or events to which they are already attending.

Toddlers with Down syndrome are less interested in toys and other objects than typically developing toddlers are, and spend more time in mutual eye gaze with their caregivers (Kaiser et al., 2001). Thus, it is especially important for adults to introduce situations in which children are likely to become engaged with desirable objects and then provide appropriate linguistic input while maintaining joint attention. If the child does not spontaneously attend to any of the available objects, then the adult should choose an object that he or she thinks is likely to be of particular interest to the child and then try to focus the child's attention on that object.

As part of these episodes of joint attention, it is critical to establish turn taking with the child. Initially, the child's turn may be nonverbal. As the child's expressive language develops, turns should increasingly become verbal. Children with Down syndrome take longer to process verbal input than typically developing children do and also take more time to formulate their response. Thus, it is critical that the adults interacting with the child with Down syndrome allow the child more time to take his or her turn than they would allow a typically developing child. Chapman (1999) suggests a wait time of three seconds between when the adult finishes his or her turn and when a response is expected from the child with Down syndrome. Initially, waiting this long may feel awkward for the adult, but as the child begins to take his or her turn regularly, the adult will find this extended wait time more and more comfortable.

Maintaining a comfortable and effective communicative environment: choosing objects, object labels, and communication modalities

As the research reviewed earlier in this chapter indicated, the onset of expressive oral language is often extremely delayed for children with Down syndrome and the rate of progress after the child begins to talk typically is very slow. To increase the rate at which children learn to communicate linguistically, sign language is often introduced in conjunction with oral language ('total communication'). Ideally input composed of simultaneous speech and sign is provided, starting during the prelinguistic period. Parents may learn signs from books or videotapes, although a brief sign language course, ideally geared to parents of young children, is quite helpful. Launonen (1996) compared the impact of input composed of keyword signing (signing only the most important words in an utterance) plus speech to that of input composed of speech alone, with regard to increases in total expressive vocabulary size, primary form of communication, and more general aspects of development. Two years after the intervention ended, children in the keyword signing group had significantly larger expressive vocabularies, were more likely to use speech as their primary form of linguistic communication, and had more advanced cognitive, social, and adaptive development than the speech only group. This project, along with a series of case studies, demonstrates the value of signed input for children with Down syndrome. (See Clibbens, 2001, for a review.)

For signed input to be effective, it must occur within the context of joint attention, ideally to the child's ongoing focus of attention. Clibbens, Powell and Atkinson (2002) have identified two effective strategies based on studies of deaf signers interacting with their deaf infants and toddlers. First, the adult may reach around the child to sign in his or her signing space. Second, the adult may displace signs that are typically made on the speaker's body to the child's body. Clibbens et al. suggest that the use of displaced signing would increase the rate at which children learn contact signs (a type of sign that is particularly difficult to teach).

In addition to providing simultaneous speech and signed input in the context of joint attention to a focus chosen by the child, it is important to choose carefully the labels that will be used and the exemplars to be labelled. As mentioned earlier in this chapter, objects may be labelled at a variety of different hierarchical levels. Children learn basic-level names for objects (for example, 'dog') much more easily than either superordinate names (such as 'animal') or subordinate ones (such as 'collie'), so it is most effective to label objects at this level. Felicitously, naming at this level is natural for most adults when talking with young children. For children who are just beginning to acquire language, labels are best provided as part of short phrases or sentences, with the label at the end of the utterance (to take advantage of the recency effect in short-term memory). Furthermore, at this stage of lexical development children need to hear a word multiple times, on multiple occasions, with the referent clearly identified before they are able to map it to the appropriate referent. Thus, it is important to label an object with the same word several times as part of each interaction. Early in the acquisition process, the task of mapping a word to its referent is so difficult for the child that he or she is likely to attempt this process only for objects or events that he or she finds especially motivating. Thus it is important to choose carefully the child's toys or other objects with which he or she interacts, to maximize the child's motivation to learn the names for these objects. Taking the child on outings where he or she is likely to see objects of interest (for example, zoo, farm, construction site, hardware store) offers focused opportunities for providing input regarding particularly motivating objects. It also is important that the initial exemplars labelled be good examples of their category (for instance, for *bird*, a robin rather than a penguin) and that they are real objects or realistic replicas or pictures, rather than stylistic objects or pictures.

Once the child begins to produce labels (either signed, spoken, or both), it is likely that the range of referents to which he or she applies a given label will not be identical to that for an adult. In some of these cases, the label used by the child will be clearly incorrect (for example, calling a boat, 'airplane') and may well be a performance error. In such cases, it is appropriate for the adult to provide the correct label in an unobtrusive manner. In many cases, however, the child's label will correspond to the expected child-basic category (for example, labelling a tiger, 'kitty' or a spherical candle, 'ball'). In these cases, it is best to accept the child's label until the adult thinks the child is able to appreciate the attributes that differentiate the object from other members of its child-basic category. At that time, the adult-basic label may be introduced using the label plus verbal description and concrete illustration of differentiating attributes method described earlier in this chapter. It is important to remember that even after the child begins to comprehend the adult-basic label for an object that previously was included in a child-basic category of a different name, the child may continue also to include the object in the child-basic category. This is a normal developmental phase. A critical goal of language intervention is for the child to enjoy talking (or signing) and to discover the power of words (signs). Supporting the child's use of child-basic labels until he or she is ready to learn adult-basic labels is an important component of demonstrating to the child the effectiveness of language for communication.

In conclusion, although children with Down syndrome typically have significant difficulty with language acquisition, there is both a great deal of variability in language ability across individuals with Down syndrome and also important steps that can be taken to facilitate language growth. Providing simultaneous oral and signed input within the context of joint attention is critical. Such input will be most effective if it is produced regarding objects or events on which the child has chosen to focus his or her attention, rather than objects or events selected by the adult. Objects or actions will need to be labelled multiple times, on multiple occasions, before children just starting to acquire language will be able to learn their names. Referents should be realistic, representative exemplars of their category, which the child finds intrinsically motivating. Support of child-basic labels until the child is ready to learn adult-basic labels is critical for demonstrating to the child the utility of words (signs) for communication. Sufficient wait time should be provided to afford the child an opportunity to take his or her turn before the adult answers for the child. It is important, within this type of interaction structure, that adults talk with children as much as possible; Huttenlocher (1998) has shown that the amount of input provided to a child has a major impact on his or her rate of vocabulary development. In turn, rate of vocabulary development influences rate of syntactic development (Bates and Goodman, 1997). Furthermore, at least for children with Down syndrome, rate of early vocabulary development, once vocabulary acquisition has begun, is strongly related not only to later verbal ability but also to later nonverbal ability (Mervis, Robinson, and Bertrand, 1998) and thus likely plays a major role in functioning even during adulthood.

References

Baddeley AD, Gathercole S, Papagno C (1998) The phonological loop as a language learning device. Psychological Review 105: 158–73.

Bates E, Goodman J (1997) On the inseparability of grammar and the lexicon: evidence from acquisition aphasia and real-time processing. Language and Cognitive Processes 12: 507–86.

Berglund E, Eriksson M, Johansson I (2001) Parental reports of spoken language skills in children with Down syndrome. Journal of Speech, Language, and Hearing Research 44: 179–91.

Beeghly M, Cicchetti D (1997) Talking about self and other: Emergence of an internal state lexicon in young children with Down syndrome. Development and Psychopathology 9: 729–48.

Bloom L (2000) The intentionality model of word learning: How to learn a word, any word. In Golinkoff RM, Hirsh-Pasek K, Bloom L, Smith LB, Woodward, AL, Akhtar N, Tomasello M, Hollich G (eds) Becoming a Word Learner: A debate on lexical Acquisition. Oxford: Oxford University Press, pp. 19–50.

Cardoso-Martins C, Mervis CB, Mervis CA (1985) Early vocabulary acquisition by children with Down syndrome. American Journal of Mental Deficiency 90: 177–84.

Carey S (1978) The child as word learner. In M Halle, J Bresnan, GA Miller (eds) Linguistic Theory and Psychological Reality. Cambridge Mass: MIT Press, pp. 264–93.

Carpenter M, Nagell K, Tomasello M (1998) Social cognition, joint attention, and communicative competence from 9 to 15 months of age. Monographs of the Society for Research in Child Development 63 (4, Serial No. 255).

Caselli MC, Vicari S, Longobardi E, Lami L, Pizzoli C, Stella G (1998) Gestures and words in early development of children with Down syndrome. Journal of Speech, Language, and Hearing Research 41: 1125–35.

Chapman R, Kay-Raining Bird E, Schwartz S (1990) Fast mapping of words in event context by children with Down syndrome. Journal of Speech and Hearing Disorders 55: 761–70.

Chapman R (1999) Language development in children and adolescents with Down syndrome. In J Miller, M Leddy, LA Leavitt (eds) Improving the Communication of People with Down Syndrome. Baltimore Md: Brookes, pp. 41–60.

Clibbens J (2001) Signing and lexical development in children with Down syndrome. Down Syndrome Research and Practice 7: 101–5.

Clibbens J, Powell GC, Atkinson E (2002) Strategies for achieving joint attention when signing to children with Down syndrome. International Journal of Language and Communication Disorders 37: 309–23.

Corrigan R (1978) Language development as related to stage six object permanence development. Journal of Child Language 5: 173–89.

Dale PS, Fenson L (1996) Lexical development norms for young children. Behavioral Research Methods, Instruments, and Computers 28: 125–7.

Dunn J, Brown J (1991) Relationships, talk about feelings, and the development of affect regulation in early childhood. In J Garber, KA Dodge (eds) The Development of Emotion Regulation and Dysregulation. New York: Cambridge University Press, pp. 89–108.

Fenson L, Dale PS, Reznick JS, Thal D, Bates E, Hartung JP, Pethick S, Reilly JS (1993) MacArthur Communicative Development Inventories: User's Guide and Technical Manual. San Diego Calif: Singular Press.

Fenson L, Dale PS, Reznick JS, Bates E, Thal D, Pethick S (1994) Variability in early communicative development. Monographs of the Society for Research in Child Development, 59 (5, Serial No. 242).

Folger MK, Leonard LB (1978) Language and sensorimotor development during the early period of referential speech. Journal of Speech and Hearing Research 21: 518–27.

Franco F, Wishart JG (1995) Use of pointing and other gestures by young children with Down syndrome. American Journal on Mental Retardation 100: 160–82.

Gillham B (1979) The First Words Language Programme: a Basic Language Programme for Mentally Handicapped Children. London: George Allen & Unwin.

Girolametto L, Weitzman E, Clements-Baartman J (1998) Vocabulary intervention for children with Down syndrome: Parent training using focused stimulation. Infant-toddler Intervention: The Transdisciplinary Journal 8: 109–25.

Greenwald CA, Leonard LB (1979) Communicative and sensorimotor development of Down's syndrome children. American Journal on Mental Deficiency 84: 296–303.

Harris S, Kasari C, Sigman M (1996) Joint attention and language gains in children with Down syndrome. Journal on Mental Retardation 100: 608–19.

Huttenlocher J (1998) Language input and language growth. Preventative Medicine 27: 195–9.

Jarrold C, Baddeley AD, Phillips C (1999) Down syndrome and the phonological loop: the evidence for, and importance of, a specific verbal short-term memory deficit. Down Syndrome Research and Practice 6: 61–75.

Kaiser AP, Hester PP, McDuffie AS (2001) Supporting communication in young children with developmental disabilities. Mental Retardation and Developmental Disabilities Research Reviews 7: 143–50.

Kay-Raining Bird E, Gaskell A, Dallaire Babineau M, MacDonald S (2000) Novel word acquisition in children with Down syndrome: does modality make a difference? Journal of Communication Disorders 33: 241–66.

Kumin L, Councill C, Goodman M (1998) Expressive vocabulary development in children with Down syndrome. Down Syndrome Quarterly 3: 1–7.

Kumin L, Councill C, Goodman M (1999) Expressive vocabulary in young children with Down syndrome: from research to treatment. Infant-Toddler Intervention: The Transdisciplinary Journal 9: 87–100.

Launonen K (1996) Enhancing communicative skills of children with Down syndrome: Early use of manual signs. In S von Techner, MH Jenson (eds) Augmentative and Alternative Communications: European Perspectives. London: Whurr.

Masur EF (1982). Mother's responses to infants' object-related gestures: influences on lexical development. Journal of Child Language 9: 23–30.

Mervis CB (1983) Acquisition of a lexicon. Contemporary Educational Psychology 8: 210–36.

Mervis CB (1984) Early lexical development: the contributions of mother and child. In C Sophian (ed.) Origins of Cognitive Skills. Hillsdale NJ: Erlbaum, pp. 339–70.

Mervis CB (1987) Child-basic object categories and early lexical development. In U Neisser (ed.) Concepts and Conceptual Development: Ecological and Intellectual Factors in Categorization. Cambridge: Cambridge University Press, pp. 201–33.

Mervis CB (1990) Early conceptual development of children with Down syndrome. In D Cicchetti, M Beeghly (eds) Children with Down Syndrome: A Developmental Perspective. Cambridge: Cambridge University Press, pp. 252–301.

Mervis CB, Bertrand J (1994) Acquisition of the Novel Name-Nameless Category (N3C) principle. Child Development 65: 1646–62.

Mervis CB, Bertrand J (1995) Acquisition of the Novel Name-Nameless Category (N3C) principle by young children who have Down syndrome. American Journal of Mental Retardation 100: 231–43.

Mervis CB, Bertrand J (1997) Developmental relations between cognition and language: evidence from Williams syndrome. In LB Adamson, MA Romski (eds) Communication and Language Acquisition: Discoveries from Atypical Development. Baltimore Md: Brookes, pp. 75–106.

Mervis CB, Mervis CA, Johnson KE, Bertrand J (1992) Studying early lexical development: the value of the systematic diary method. In C Rovee-Collier, L Lipsitt (eds) Advances in Infancy Research. Norwood NJ: Ablex, vol. 7, pp. 291–378.

Mervis CB, Pani JR, Pani AM (in press) Transaction of child cognitive-linguistic abilities and adult input in the acquisition and evolution of lexical categories at the basic and subordinate levels. In DH Rakison, LM Oakes (eds) Early Category and Concept Development. Oxford: Oxford University Press.

Mervis CB, Robinson BF (2000) Expressive vocabulary ability of toddlers with Williams syndrome or Down syndrome: a comparison. Developmental Neuropsychology 17: 111–26.

Mervis CB, Robinson BF, Bertrand J (1998. Vocabulary growth curves of children with Williams syndrome or Down syndrome. Gatlinburg Conference on Research and Theory in Mental Retardation and Developmental Disabilities, Charlestown, SC, March.

Miller JF (1992) Lexical development in young children with Down syndrome. In R Chapman (ed.) Processes in Language Acquisition and Disorders. St Louis Mo: Mosby, pp. 202–16.

Miller JF (1999) Profiles of language development in children with Down syndrome. In JF Miller, M Leddy, LA Leavitt (eds) Improving the Communication of People with Down Syndrome. Baltimore Md: Brookes, pp. 11–39.

Miller JF, Sedey AL, Miolo G (1995) Validity of parent report measures of vocabulary development for children with Down syndrome. Journal of Speech and Hearing Research 38: 1037–44.

Mundy P, Kasari C, Sigman M, Ruskin E (1995) Nonverbal communication and early language acquisition in children with Down syndrome and in normally developing children. Journal of Speech and Hearing Research 38: 157–67.

Nelson K (1973) Structure and strategy in learning to talk. Monographs of the Society for Research in Child Development 38 (1–2, Serial No. 149).

Oliver B, Buckley S (1994) The language development of children with Down's syndrome: first words to two word phrases. Down's Syndrome: Research and Practice 2: 71–5.

Rondal JA (1995) Exceptional language development in Down syndrome. New York: Cambridge University Press.

Rosch E, Mervis CB, Gray WD, Johnson DM, Boyes-Braem P (1976) Basic objects in natural categories. Cognitive Psychology 8: 382–439.

Sigman M, Ruskin E (1999) Continuity and change in the social competence of children with autism, Down syndrome, and developmental delays. Monographs of the Society for Research in Child Development, 64, Serial no. 256.

Singer Harris N, Bellugi U, Bates E, Jones W, Rossen M (1997) Contrasting profiles of language development in children with Williams and Down syndromes. Developmental Neuropsychology 13: 345–70.

Smith L, von Techner S, Michalsen B (1998) The emergence of language skills in young children with Down syndrome. In L Nadel (ed.) The Psychobiology of Down Syndrome. Cambridge Mass: Bradford Press, pp. 145–65.

Tomasello M, Farrar MJ (1986) Joint attention and early language. Child Development 57: 1454–63.

Tomasello M (2001) Perceiving intentions and learning words in the second year of life. In M Bowerman, SC Levinson (eds) Language Acquisition and Conceptual Development. Cambridge: Cambridge University Press, pp. 132–58.

Vallar G, Papagno C (1993) Preserved vocabulary acquisition in Down's syndrome: the role of phonological short-term memory. Cortex 29: 467–83.

Vicari S, Caselli MC, Tonucci F (2000) Asynchrony of lexical and morphosyntactic development in children with Down syndrome. Neuropsychologia 38: 634–44.

Acknowledgement

Preparation of this manuscript was supported by grant #HD29957 from the National Institute of Child Health and Human Development. Correspondence regarding this chapter should be addressed to Carolyn Mervis, Dept. of Psychological and Brain Sciences, University of Louisville, Louisville, KY 40292 USA or cbmervis@louisville.edu.

Chapter 6
Morphosyntactic training and intervention

JEAN A RONDAL

Semantic or thematic relations or structures are the building blocks on which grammatical (or more exactly morphosyntactic) development takes place. As might be expected, individuals with intellectual disabilities are delayed in thematic semantic development in proportion to their cognitive deficit.

Semantic structural development

When they begin to combine two and three words within the same utterance (often not before 3 to 4 years, chronological age), children with Down syndrome appear to express the same range of relational meanings or thematic roles and relations as reported by the students of early combinatorial language in the typically developing child, and pertaining to the semantic structures of the natural languages. Examples of early thematic relations expressed both by typically developing children and children with intellectual disabilities are notice or existence, denial, disappearance, recurrence, attribution, possession, location, instrument, conjunction, agent–action, action–object, and agent–action–object. Fowler, Gelman, and Gleitman (1994) recorded spontaneous speech samples for children with Down syndrome (chronological age range 10; 9 to 13 years) matched for mean length of utterance (MLU) with younger typically developing children. The children's MLUs were in the range 2.75 to 3.25 words plus inflectional morphemes (mean 2.98). The researchers reported that children in both groups were explicit in expressing most of the obligatory thematic relations studied in early language development. Non-stative verbs and stative locative verbs (for example, 'sit', 'belong') were expressed virtually 100% of the time. Stative verbs were often implicit as they are in typically developing children early in semantic structural development (Bloom, Miller and Hood, 1975). For example, children with Down syndrome frequently produced utterances such as 'the doll upstairs', while placing a doll in a doll's house, implying a verb such as 'belongs'. Overall, obligatory nominal arguments entering into locative relations were supplied 72% of the time by children with Down syndrome and 75% of the time by the typically developing group. The most important tendency was to omit an obligatory nominal element involving the agent (in grammatical subject role) of agent locative utterances, as in 'put it here'. Individuals with Down syndrome omitted this constituent 61% of the time in average value versus 25% in the typically developing group. However, sentence subjects were most consistently supplied when functioning as patients in locative state utterances (for example, 'tyres belong in the garage'). Children with Down syndrome consistently supplied the patient in object position (76% in average score) versus 95% in the typically developing group.

There is no indication that the semantic structural basis of combinatorial language, as it is put to use in early language production and reception, is markedly different in children with Down syndrome and typically developing children at corresponding levels of language development.

Morphosyntactic development

Morphosyntactic development is slow and remains largely incomplete in individuals with Down syndrome. Some progress is obvious with increased chronological age, at least until early adolescence. This progress is illustrated in MLU measures. Most often, children with Down syndrome reach MLU 2 around 4 to 5 years chronological age, MLU 3 around 7 to 8 years, and MLU 6 around 14 or 15 years. They plateau definitively or with very little progress beyond this level. In comparison, typically developing children reach MLU 5 or more around 6 years.

The slowness and limitation of MLU development in children with Down syndrome correspond to important shortcomings in morphosyntax. Word order in those languages relying on sequential devices to express thematic relations (such as English and French) is usually correct, however (Rondal, 1978a,b, 1985; Rosenberg and Abbeduto, 1993; Lomonte, 1995). There is a paradox here. Children with Down syndrome do not seem to have particular problems with word order in simple utterances whereas they often have serious difficulties with other morphosyntactic aspects of language. Why should word order be spared in intellectual disabilities? It will not suffice to say that word order is a simpler matter to master than other grammatical devices. We know that word ordering has to be learned and is in no way a simple matter. It is not obvious why it should be easier to process than grammatical morphology. No explanation is available to the best of my knowledge regarding this paradox.

In young children with Down syndrome, the production of grammatical words (functors) is reduced (the articles, prepositions, pronouns, modals, auxiliaries, copula and conjunctions). This gives the utterances of these children a telegraphic character. Later in development, as indicated by data collected by Fowler et al. (1994), the proportions of pronouns, prepositions, modals, WH-forms and demonstratives are similar in Down syndrome and MLU-matched typically developing children. The same children with Down syndrome supplied overall percentages of grammatical morphemes, which were virtually identical to those of MLU-matched typically developing children (around 66%). There were some differences, however, regarding the patterns of acquisition for individual morphemes. Children with Down syndrome were more variable in their production. Rutter and Buckley (1994) reported (based on parental reports) that most morphemes among the major ones had been acquired at least by some of their subjects, in the same order as the one reported for typically developing children, and that the acquisition delay varied between 3 and 15 months-chronological age. The following morphemes were not mastered, however; noncontracted copula 'be', third person singular marking on verb, and noncontracted auxiliary 'be'. Chapman, Schwartz and Kay-Raining Bird (1992) (see also Chapman, 1995) observed that older children with Down syndrome and adolescents more frequently omit free and bound grammatical morphemes than MLU-matched typically developing controls in narrative speech samples. Similarly, Bol and Kuiken (1990) documented fewer verb agreements and less frequent use of pronouns in the language of Dutch children with Down syndrome with a chronological age of 8 to 19 years (MAs greater than 3 years and 6 months), when compared to that of typically developing children aged 1 to 4 years. It seems clear that, despite some variation in the data (probably, at least partially linked to individual variation), individuals with Down syndrome have persistent difficulties with the grammatical morphemes.

Fowler et al. (1994) also computed several syntactic measures on their cross-sectional samples of spontaneous speech from children with Down syndrome. They were making little use of complex constructions, such as passives, subject/auxiliary inversions and conjoined clauses. Multi-verb utterances were rare, comprising fewer than 5% of the utterances. One particular child with Down syndrome, named Rebecca, was followed longitudinally between 50 and 89 months of age. Rebecca's syntactic evolution was reported to parallel that of younger typically developing children regarding early negative and interrogative constructions. Beyond 67 months, however, she failed to make further syntactic progress. The auxiliary system underlying mature negative and interrogative sentences was almost totally lacking in her grammar. She would make persistent overuse of the term 'what' in order to introduce most 'wh-' questions. The 'what' term largely replaced other 'wh-' terms such as 'when', 'where' and 'how'. Correspondingly, Jenny, the 6-year-old child with Down syndrome studied cross-sectionally by Michaelis (1976) was reported not to produce 'wh-' questions.

The above studies confirm previous reports (for example, Lenneberg, Nichols and Rosenberger, 1964; Lackner, 1968; Rondal, 1978a) on the important problems individuals with intellectual disabilities have with syntactic aspects of expressive language, and their increasing delay compared with mental age-matched typically developing controls.

There are also numerous reports pointing to the serious limitations of children and adolescents with Down syndrome in the comprehension of morphosyntactic structures. They lag behind mental age-matched typically developing controls in this respect too (see Rondal, 1975, 1985; Rondal and Edwards, 1997 for reviews).

Kernan (1990) has documented the difficulty of young adults with moderate or mild intellectual disabilities (Down syndrome and intellectual disabilities of unidentified etiology) in processing temporal sentences. Both samples of subjects exhibited patterns of comprehension that resembled those of younger typically developing children. Sentences that referred to temporally related events with clause order matching the order in which the events happened, were happening, or would be happening, proved easier to process by the individuals with intellectual disabilities. This was the case for the following types of sentences:

- 'X then Y' (for example 'The dog jumps over the cat and then the cat jumps over the dog.')
- 'X before Y' ('John sat down before Mary sat down.')
- 'After X, Y' (for example 'After the cat jumped over the dog, the dog jumped over the cat.')

Sentences in which the clause order did not match the order of the events (for example, 'before X, Y' and 'X after Y' sentences) yielded markedly lower proportions of correct interpretative answers.

Comblain, Fayasse and Rondal (1993) found children, adolescents and adults with Down syndrome performing markedly poorer than typically developing children on the Batterie d'Evaluation de la Morpho-syntaxe (BEMS) subtests, evaluating the comprehension of personal pronouns, definite and indefinite articles, subordinate clauses, negative and passive sentences. Corresponding data have been obtained by Fayasse, Comblain, and Rondal (1995). They administered the BEMS to a group of French-speaking children, adolescents and young adults who were typically developing or had mild or moderate intellectual disabilities. Results of the analyses confirm the existence of remarkable similarities in the hierarchies of difficulty of the grammatical structures proposed, the types of errors observed and the developmental sequences across the groups of subjects, despite marked differences between the groups in absolute frequencies of errors (favouring typically developing individuals and individuals with mild intellectual disabilities, as expected). Classifying the receptive tasks on the BEMS according to increasing order of difficulty yielded the same sequences for typically developing individuals and for individuals with mild and moderate intellectual disabilities. Spearman rank correlation coefficients computed on the hierarchies of grammatical difficulty revealed significant associations between the groups of subjects. Such data are supportive of the continuity hypothesis in grammatical development and functioning between individuals with typical development and those with intellectual disabilities on the one hand, and between levels of intellectual disabilities on the other.

Voice in the sentence processing of individuals with intellectual disabilities has been dealt with systematically in few studies. Rondal, Cession, and Vincent (1988) studied the comprehension of declarative mono-propositional sentences varying according to voice and semantic transitivity features (see Hopper and Thompson, 1980) in a group of 17 young adults with Down syndrome. They were tested for comprehension of a set of plausible and (thematic or event) reversible active and passive declarative sentences. Kinesis (degree of 'action-ness') of verbs was systematically varied. Subjects were requested to choose between two pictures. One picture correctly represented the thematic relation encoded in the sentence heard (for example, girl pushing boy, for the sentence 'The girl pushes the boy.') The other picture corresponded to a reversal of the same relation (for example, boy pushing girl, for the same sentence).

Passive sentences do not differ from active ones in the thematic relations expressed but only in the overt realization of these relations. Passive sentences have their underlying logical subject realized in the surface form of an oblique object most often introduced by the preposition by (for example, 'the boy' in the sentence 'The girl was pushed by the boy.') Their underlying logical object is realized in the form of the surface subject – 'the girl' in the sentence above). Typically developing children understand active as well as passive sentences earlier and better when the sentences are constructed around actions verbs (for example 'push', 'carry') – verbs taking agent as subjects, as opposed to mental verbs (for example, 'imagine', 'like', 'see') (Rondal, Thibaut and Cession, 1990). In line with the work of Kosslyn (1980) and Paivio (1986), Rondal et al. (1990) suggested that the action verb effect could be due to a particular supporting role of the mental image to the computations involved in sentence processing, especially when the analytic task is more complex or with certain types of formal structures; the construction of a mental image being favoured in the case of concrete and action verbs. This hypothesis was corroborated in a study by Thibaut, Rondal, and Kaens (1995) on the role of mental imagery in sentence comprehension. The experimental results obtained by Rondal et al. (1988) indicate that the facilitating effect of kinesis is as true of the adults with Down syndrome studied as it is of typically developing children, except that with the former the effect is limited to active sentences. Adults with Down syndrome with relatively higher IQs (range 40 to 60) correctly interpreted 83% of the action-verb active sentences versus 73% of the nonaction ones. Adults with Down syndrome with relatively lower IQs (range 20 to 39) obtained 75% and 50% correct interpretation, respectively. For the nonaction verb passives, the profiles of responses also differed according to IQ level. The higher IQ group interpreted passive sentences as if they were corresponding actives in 60% of the cases versus 70% for the lower IQ group. The action-verb passives were interpreted at chance level in the two groups (50% and 47% for the higher and the lower IQ groups, respectively).

This research shows, first, that in a large majority of cases, adults with Down syndrome do not correctly understand the morphosyntactic and semantic aspects associated with the passive voice and, second, that the reversible declarative active sentences are correctly understood in a good proportion of the cases, particularly when action verbs are used and at higher IQ levels. For active sentences, therefore, the same facilitating effect of semantic kinesis can be shown in adults with Down syndrome as in typically developing children. It may be supposed that the structural complexity of the passive not only makes problems of comprehension for individuals with Down syndrome, but also blocks potentially facilitating semantic actionality effects.

Using the same picture-designating technique as Rondal et al. (1988), Comblain (1989) confirmed that adults with Down syndrome, as a group, interpret reversible passive sentences with action or non-action verbs at chance level or below. One aspect of Comblain's work deserves additional consideration. She presented her subjects with series of monopropositional active and passive sentences randomly mixing plausible (for example 'the boy hits the girl') and implausible statements (for example, 'le vélo est détesté par le livre' – 'the bike is hated by the book'). Treating such series of sentences, the adults with Down syndrome – but not the typically developing adults constituting the control group – also interpreted the actives at or near chance level. This shows how relatively fragile and semantic-pragmatically dependent even the linguistic treatment of simple active declarative sentences may remain in DS individuals.

Discursive development

Limited information is available on the discursive capacities of individuals with Down syndrome. Reilly, Klima and Bellugi (1991) compared cognitively matched adolescents with Williams syndrome or Down syndrome in a story-telling activity. The teenagers were introduced to a wordless picture book, *Frog, Where are You?* They were asked to tell a story from the pictures as they progressed page by page through the book. In contrast with individuals with Down syndrome, the adolescents with Williams syndrome told coherent and complex narratives that made extensive use of affective prosody. The teenagers with Williams syndrome, but not those with Down syndrome, enriched the referential contents of their stories with narrative, affective and social cognitive devices. For example, those with Williams syndrome used markedly more features such as affective and mental verbs, emphatic and intensifier forms, negative markers, causal connectors, as well as onomatopoeic forms.

A study by Chapman, Schwartz and Kay-Raining Bird (1991) indirectly confirms the particular difficulty of children and adolescents with Down syndrome in online story processing. In such contexts these subjects no longer demonstrate the fast-mapping ability with novel words that they exhibit in simpler event contexts. In story contexts, individuals with Down syndrome encounter additional difficulties in processing the narrative structure and in memory for story gist generally. These difficulties interfere with inferring the likely referent of the novel words preventing the fast-mapping production forms observed in event contexts to occur. However, Chapman et al. (1992) report significant increases in the narratives of at least some older adolescents with Down syndrome in the group studied (chronological ages between 16 and 20 years) in comparison with children with Down syndrome and younger adolescents aged 5 to 16 years.

More generally, discursive functioning in persons with Down syndrome is often lacking in macrostructure organization and in cohesion. I take macrostructure here to mean the larger discursive framework in opposition to the semantic propositional and the morphosyntactic levels (discursive or textual microstructure). Discourses vary as to their basic organization. At this level it is possible to distinguish between at least, four major type of texts: narrative, argumentative, descriptive, and theoretical or explanatory (less relevant in the present context). Narratives are organized typically in chronological order. It is permissible to modify that order but the interlocutor must be duly warned (so-called markedness of the expression). By default, one will expect the speaker to start the story at the beginning and go through it chronologically, optionally terminating with a personal comment or 'moral'. Argumentative texts are not necessarily organized according to a particular chronology (although they may be). The key object here is coherence (connectedness and absence of self-contradiction). A good argument is one that is relevant and does not contradict itself. Argumentative discourses may contain several arguments. It is essential that they not only do not contradict each other but contribute each to bolster the case. Descriptive texts are not typically chronologically ordered (although, of course, they may be) and they do not need to be fully coherent (but, of course, they cannot be incoherent). Descriptive texts must obey referential adequacy – they must correspond in major ways with the objects or the events under description. The macrostructures mentioned above are clearly cognitive in nature and as such can be expected to make problems for people with intellectual disabilities. Such is also the case most often for textual cohesion. According to Halliday (1985), textual cohesion is realized by four major ways:

- *Reference:* a participant or circumstantial element introduced at one place in the text can be taken as a reference point for something that follows (for example, 'the boy . . . he . . . him' – pronominal use, in such cases, implies correct application of the coreference rule between noun and pronoun (see Appendix 1, under 'pronouns').
- *Ellipsis:* a clause or part of a clause once formulated may be presupposed and omitted at a subsequent place in text.
- *Lexical cohesion:* discursive continuity may also be established by the choice of words that may take the form of word repetition, the presence of key words, or the choice of words that are related semantically to previous ones.
- *Conjunction:* a clause or some longer portion of text may be related to what follows by one of a set of particular words (adverbs, conjunctions) carrying relational or hierarchical meaning (for example, 'then', 'in such a way as', 'therefore', 'but', 'because', 'for').

The above cohesive devices are often found insufficiently developed and when they are produced not always correctly used by Down syndrome persons.

Assessing morphosyntactic development

Utterance and sentence checklists can be useful (besides more formal assessment devices) as a way to follow closely and document a child's progress in the grammatical aspects of language. Regular observations (and noting) will help parents to encourage their child's ability to gradually use longer and better structured sentences. The scheme outlined in Appendix 1 is a modified and extended form of the *Sentences and Grammar Checklist* published by the Down Syndrome Educational Trust (2001). It also integrates a number of developmental indications retaken from Rondal (1986, 1997). This scheme can also be used informally to assess either the child's comprehension, production, or both (but separately).

Despite the existence of an abundant literature on language development in Down syndrome children as a group (see Rondal and Edwards, 1997, for a review) there is little precise published information regarding the rate at which individual children with Down syndrome develop morphosyntactically. However, it is known from practical and clinical experience that there are important individual differences. Some children with Down syndrome will be progressing more rapidly than others across the grammatical acquisitions outlined in Appendix 1. Although rate of progress matters (reducing developmental delays being the major objective of the intervention programmes), the gradual access of the child with Down syndrome and adolescent to more advanced grammatical levels actually is as important as the absolute time dimension in remediation.

Promoting morphosyntactic development

Comprehension (receptive) training should always precede production training for any structure to be taught. Regarding expressive training, in the first stage, the child should be encouraged to repeat words, utterances, or sentences auditorily presented in the appropriate situation. Once the child has started producing verbal material, the expansion technique should be used systematically. Expansions can be produced quite naturally in the interactive sessions with the child with Down syndrome, exactly as they are used spontaneously by parents of typical language-learning children (cf. Rondal, 1985). For example, parents and language trainers may listen carefully to the early productions of a child with Down syndrome and expand them in the shortest grammatically correct sentences. This might involve supplying the missing obligatory components of the sentence – for example:

Child: Daddy gone.
Adult: Daddy has gone.

Child: Cat sleeping.
Adult: The cat is sleeping.

Child: Mummy go car.
Adult: Mummy has gone out in the car.

Child: Play sand.
Adult: Can I play in the sand, please?

Child: Daddy go work.
Adult: Daddy is going to work.

It is not necessary that the child correctly repeats at once the expanded forms proposed by the adult, not even that he or she tries to repeat it in any way. In the long term, however, expanding children utterances into more complex structures will pay off in the sense that the child, including the child with Down syndrome, will gradually incorporate the grammatical material into his or her spontaneous productions.

Direct and explicit corrections should be avoided particularly with the younger child. Only with the older child, adolescent, or young adult, could more direct explicit modelling and corrections be used as a secondary way helping to promote better grammatical language in persons with Down syndrome.

The developmental indications summarized in Appendix 1 will be useful in guiding not only the professional and the educated parents to follow closely the grammatical development of children with Down syndrome but also in guiding remediation efforts as to this target. It is indicated to expand the child's production with an eye, so to speak, to the grammatical development scheme, having in mind the next step(s) that the child is going to negotiate as opposed to trying to reach too far at a given time, rendering things more difficult for the child and his or her trainer. Here, the Vygotskyian notion of 'zone of proximal development' should guide the trainers' remediation efforts, ensuring that what is expected from and proposed to the child at a given time (step) in development always is precisely located within immediate reach from the previous acquisition. This, of course, supposes that the development can be in some way specified longitudinally with some minimal degree of precision, which I have tried to do in a summary way in the preceding pages (for a more detailed and precise treatment and developmental analysis, see Rondal and Edwards, 1997).

Regarding the scheme proposed in Appendix 1, it should be kept in mind that the 'more advanced morphosyntactic structures' should be considered optional for many Down syndrome persons and not at all as an obligatory developmental or remediation course.

It should be noted also that, as shown in research (cf. Rondal, 1978a; Rondal and Edwards, 1997; Marfo, Dedrick and Barbour, 1998), the parents of children with intellectual disabilities or Down syndrome, as a group, spontaneously interact linguistically with their children in the same way as parents of typically developing children do with their own children at corresponding language levels. The purpose, therefore, of involving parents in the language remediation of their own children with Down syndrome is not to teach them how to interact communicatively with their children – they do it quite properly, as a rule – but, instead, to optimize their language relationship with their children in the perspective of remediation by going beyond the spontaneous adaptation to language-learning children (even if delayed) towards systematic modelling of correct morphosyntactic structures and expanding on children's productions as a way to foster accelerated development in children with Down syndrome.

A last point to consider is the existence of a critical period for morphosyntactic development in those with typical development as well as those with intellectual disabilities. As argued by Hurford (1991), the main determinant for the ending time parameters of the critical periods are the evolutionary consequences of the interplay of genetic factors influencing life-history characteristics in relation to language acquisition. If this is so, there is no way that those with intellectual disabilities or Down syndrome can escape the critical periodical constraints. Lenneberg (1967), Fowler (1988) and Fowler et al. (1994) have indeed claimed that language development in individuals with intellectual disabilities slows down and comes to a stop some time after puberty. However, the extensive data analysis carried out by Rondal and Edwards (1997) leads to a more complex conclusion. There does seem to be little spontaneous progress beyond mid-adolescence in the phonological and morphosyntactic aspects of language but one may witness some progress in some subjects in the lexical, pragmatic and communicative aspects, even if limited in scope, until early adulthood and sometimes beyond.

The implication regarding grammatical training with persons with Down syndrome is clear: do as much of it as is possible before mid-adolescence, for no matter how clever the intervention programme, the results in that area may largely depend on the person's brain maturational calendar.

References

Bloom L, Miller P, Hood L (1975) Variation as aspect of competence in language development. In A Pick (ed.) Minnesota Symposium on Child Language. Minneapolis Minn: University of Minnesota Press, pp. 3–55.

Bol G, Kuiken F (1990) Grammatical analysis of developmental language disorders: a study of the morphosyntax of children with specific language disorders, with hearing impairment and with Down's syndrome. Clinical Linguistics and Phonetics 4: 77–86.

Chapman R (1995) Language development in children and adolescents with Down's syndrome. In P Fletcher, B McWhinney (eds) The Handbook of Child Language. Oxford: Blackwell, pp. 641–63.

Chapman R, Schwartz S, Kay-Raining Bird E (1991) Language skills of children and adolescents with Down's syndrome: I. Comprehension. Journal of Speech and Hearing Research 34: 1106–1120.

Chapman R, Schwartz S, Kay-Raining Bird E (1992) Language production of children and adolescents with Down's Syndrome. Paper presented at the 9th World Congress of the International Association for the Scientific Study of Mental Deficiency, Gold Coast, Australia, August.

Comblain A (1989) Compréhension de la voix passive chez l'adulte trisomique 21. Master's thesis, University of Liège, Belgium (unpublished).

Comblain A, Fayasse M, Rondal JA (1993) Batterie d'évaluation morphosyntaxique (BEMS). Experimental version. University of Liège, Belgium (unpublished).

Down Syndrome Educational Trust (2001) The Down Syndrome Resources and Activities. Sentences and Grammar Check List. Appendix. Portsmouth: The Sarah Duffen Center, p. 112.

Fayasse M, Comblain A, Rondal JA (1995) Compréhension et production des classes formelles et des structures phrasiques chez les enfants et adolescents retardés mentaux. Research report. University of Liège, Laboratory for Psycholinguistics (unpublished).

Fowler A (1988) Determinants of rate of language growth in children with Down's syndrome. In L Nadel (ed.) The Psychobiology of Down's syndrome. Cambridge Mass: MIT Press, pp. 217–45.

Fowler A, Gelman R, Gleitman L (1994) The course of language learning in children with Down's syndrome. In H Tager-Flusberg (ed.), Constraints on Language Acquisition. Studies of Atypical Children. Hillsdale NJ: Erlbaum, pp. 91–140.

Halliday M (1985) An Introduction to Functional Grammar. London: Arnold.

Hopper P, Thompson S (1980) Transitivity in grammar and discourse. Language 56: 251–99.

Hurford J (1991).The evolution of the critical period for language acquisition. Cognition 40: 159–201.

Kernan K (1990) Comprehension of syntactically indicated sequence by Down's syndrome and other mentally retarded adults. Journal of Mental Deficiency Research 34: 169–78.

Kosslyn S (1980) Image and mind. Cambridge Mass: Harvard University Press.

Lackner J (1968) A developmental study of language behavior in retarded children. Neuropsychologist 6: 301–20.

Lenneberg E (1967) Biological foundations of language. New York: Wiley.

Lenneberg E, Nichols I, Rosenberger E (1964) Primitive steps of language development in mongolism. In D McRioch and E Weinstein (eds) Disorders of Communication. Baltimore Md: Williams and Wilkins, pp. 119–37.

Lomonte V (1995) Acquisition de l'ordre des mots chez l'enfant trisomique 21. Master's thesis. Universiy of Liège, Belgium (unpublished).

Marfo K, Dedrick C, Barbour N (1998) Mother–child interactions and the development of children with mental retardation. In T Burrack, R Hodapp, E Zigler (eds) Handbook of Mental Retardation and Development. New York: Cambridge University Press, pp. 637–68.

Michaelis C (1976) The language of a Down's syndrome child. Dissertation Abstracts International 37: 416.

Paivio A (1986) Mental representation: A dual-coding approach. New York: Oxford University Press.

Reilly J, Klima E, Bellugi U (1991) Once more with feeling: Affect and language in atypical populations. Developmental Psychopathology 2: 367–91.

Rondal JA (1975) Développement du langage et retard mental: une revue critique de la littérature en langue anglaise. L'Année Psychologique 75: 513–47.

Rondal J A (1978a) Maternal speech to normal and Down's syndrome children matched for mean length of utterance. In C Meyers (ed.) Quality of Life in the Severely and Profoundly Retarded People: Research Foundations for Improvement. Washington DC: American Association on Mental Deficiency, pp. 193–265.

Rondal JA (1978b) Developmental sentence scoring procedure and the delay-difference question in language development of Down's syndrome children. Mental Retardation 16: 169–171.

Rondal JA (1985) Adult–child interactions and the process of language acquisition. New York: Praeger.

Rondal JA (1986) Le développement du langage chez l'enfant trisomique 21: Manuel pratique d'aide et d'intervention. Bruxelles: Mardaga.

Rondal JA (1997) Proposal for a computer-enhaced language intervention program: cognitivo-semantico and morpho-syntactic modules. Manuscript, University of Liège, Laboratory for Psycholinguistics (unpublished).

Rondal JA, Cession A, Vincent E (1988) Compréhension des phrases déclaratives selon la voix et l'actionalité du verbe chez un groupe d'adultes trisomique 21. Manuscript, University of Liège, Laboratory for Psycholinguistics (unpublished).

Rondal JA, Edwards S (1997). Language in Mental Retardation. London: Whurr.

Rondal JA, Thibaut J, Cession A (1990) Transitivity effects on children's sentence comprehension. European Bulletin of Cognitive Psychology 10: 385–400.

Rosenberg S, Abbeduto L (1993) Language and Communication in Mental Retardation: Development, Processes, and Intervention. Hillsdale NJ: Erlbaum.

Rutter T, Buckley S (1994) The acquisition of grammatical morphemes in children with Down's syndrome. Down's Syndrome 2: 76–82.

Thibaut JP, Rondal JA, Kaens AM (1995) Actionality and mental imagery in children's comprehension of declaratives. Journal of Child Language 22: 189–209.

Chapter 7
Pragmatic development and communication training

LEONARD ABBEDUTO, YOLANDA KELLER-BELL

Language is the foundation for nearly all forms of social interaction but participating in talk with another person requires more than 'knowing' a language. It also requires the capacity to produce and understand language in real-time, goal-directed social tasks (Abbeduto and Short-Meyerson, 2002). In this chapter, we consider the challenges posed by speaking and listening for people with Down syndrome not from the perspective of their knowledge of language per se (for example, vocabulary, syntax) but rather from the perspective of their ability to use language to accomplish the social task of talking with another person. This is the domain of a field of study called *pragmatics.*

A pragmatic perspective on speaking and listening

In most current conceptualizations of pragmatics, linguistic interactions are seen as being motivated by the interpersonal goals of the participants (Abbeduto and Short-Meyerson, 2002). These goals may be as general as wanting to reminisce about 'the good old days' with a friend or as specific as wanting to learn the closing time of a new restaurant. The goals motivating an interaction typically require addressing a variety of sub-goals, such as when one must precede a request for a favour (for example, 'could you help me move out of my apartment?') by checking for potential obstacles to compliance (for example, 'are you busy on Saturday?'). Importantly, interpersonal goals can be achieved only through collaboration, which means that the behaviour of each participant in the interaction must be responsive to, and synchronized with, the behaviour, knowledge and goals of the other (Clark, 1996). Moreover, the goals of the participants typically emerge out of their personal relationships, the activities in which they are concurrently engaged, and other aspects of the context of the interaction (Abbeduto, Evans and Dolan, 2001). This means that the utterances of the participants are inextricably bound to, and can be understood only in terms of, the dynamically evolving context in which the talk is situated (Graesser, Millis and Zwaan, 1997). These conceptualizations of pragmatics lead to questions about the interpersonal goals that motivate the talk of individuals with Down syndrome, the ways in which they collaborate with a social partner to organize their behaviour and achieve their goals, the ways in which they ensure that they and their partners are understanding each other's goals as intended, and the ways in which they use context to make decisions about what to say and how to interpret what others have said. In this chapter, we consider what is known about these areas of pragmatics in persons with Down syndrome.

If speaking and listening are seen as goal-directed social activities this leads to an appreciation of the many skills and domains of functioning that are involved in, and shape, these activities (Abbeduto and Short-Meyerson, 2002). These include facility with the linguistic system, the structures and functions that comprise the human information processing system (such as auditory memory, inferential reasoning), knowledge of the objects and events that constitute the physical world, and knowledge of the human mind and the ways in which the social world is organized. Individuals with Down syndrome, as a group, have problems (relative to their same-age peers) in all of these domains of psychological and behavioural functioning, although the 'Down syndrome profile' is defined by more serious problems in some domains than in others (Abbeduto, Pavetto, Kesin, Weissman, Karadottir, O'Brien and Cawthon, 2001). This raises the question of how the Down syndrome profile shapes speaking and listening performance in real-life social interactions. In this chapter, we review what is known about the relationships between the pragmatic problems of persons with Down syndrome and their problems in other domains of behavioural and psychological functioning.

In considering what is known about the pragmatic problems of individuals with Down syndrome, we also consider the ways in which their problems differ in degree or kind from those of individuals with mental retardation due to other causes. This is not always possible, however, because researchers have not always included non-Down syndrome comparison groups in their studies. This is unfortunate because data on pragmatic problems that are specific to Down syndrome (syndrome-specific) and those that are common to individuals with mental retardation of other origins (syndrome-common) can be used to develop assessment and intervention protocols that are more closely tailored to the needs of individuals with Down syndrome. We have argued elsewhere (Abbeduto, 2001) that learning about the syndrome-specific pragmatic problems of individuals with Down syndrome will ultimately require comparison with other genetically defined groups of individuals with mental retardation, such as those with fragile X, Prader-Willi, or Williams syndrome.

Speech acts

The participants in an interaction talk to achieve interpersonal goals, such as sharing beliefs, making social contracts, obtaining information, and getting others to do one's bidding (Abbeduto and Short-Meyerson, 2002). Making these goals clear when in the role of speaker requires knowing which language forms are good candidates for expressing the desired interpersonal goal, selecting the form that will lead to the listener's recognition of the interpersonal goal in the current context, and doing the necessary 'background' work (for example, checking that the listener is attending and that he is in the 'correct' mood before asking him or her for a favour). Recognition of these linguistically expressed goals when in the role of listener requires the ability to integrate the speaker's utterance with a wide range of information from the prior discourse, the current physical and social context, and even past interactions with the other participant(s). In the field of pragmatics, these linguistically expressed interpersonal goals have typically been referred to as *speech acts* (Levinson, 1983). This is something of a misnomer, however, because many of these goals can be accomplished through nonlinguistic means, such as gestures and eye gaze. In fact, it is likely that the interpersonal goals that are the basis of speech acts have their origins in the nonverbal behavioural sequences of the prelinguistic period (Abbeduto and Hesketh, 1997). Moreover, even mature language users often rely on nonverbal behaviour for the expression of their 'speech' acts.

There is considerable evidence that typically developing children use gesture, vocalization, and eye gaze to accomplish an impressive range of 'speech' acts during the prelinguistic period (Abbeduto and Hesketh, 1997). For example, they 'request' by pointing to an object while looking urgently at an adult; they protest by pushing away an offered object and turning their face away while expressing anger or disgust; and they 'comment' by pointing and vocalizing with 'excitement' while turning back and forth between an object or event of interest and their adult partner. Researchers studying mental retardation have been interested in documenting the onset, course, and predictive power of similar nonverbally expressed speech acts in children with Down syndrome.

This research has focused largely on nonverbal 'requesting' and 'commenting' (Abbeduto and Hesketh, 1997). In two early studies, Greenwald and Leonard (1979) and Smith and Von Tetzchner (1986) studied children who were functioning at stage four or five on the Uzgiris-Hunt Scales (1975), which are a set of developmentally ordered problems thought by Piaget (1952) to reflect the important cognitive achievements of the first two years of life. These investigators focused on the maturity of the behaviours used to request and comment (for example, inclusion of both the adult partner and the object of interest within a behavioural sequence was more advanced than a behaviour that included only the adult or only the object). In both studies, it was found that the children with Down syndrome were as advanced as younger typically developing children at stage four or five at nonverbal 'requesting' but less advanced at nonverbal 'commenting'. Although children with Down syndrome use more advanced behavioural means for requesting than for commenting, they are less likely to make requests than are typically developing children or children with mental retardation of other etiologies matched to them on level of cognitive development, at least during the prelinguistic period and early stages of the linguistic period (Mundy et al., 1988, 1995).

The results of these studies suggest that Down syndrome may be characterized by substantial delays in the emergence of important nonverbally expressed interpersonal goals during the prelinguistic and early linguistic periods, and that these delays may be syndrome specific. Moreover, although there may be cognitive prerequisites for nonverbal requesting and commenting, the limitations children with Down syndrome display relative to their typically developing peers are not accounted for solely by the former group's cognitive delays. It may be that the differences between cognitively matched children with Down syndrome and typically developing children reflect broader motivational differences. For example, the less frequent requests for objects noted in children with Down syndrome by Mundy and his colleagues may reflect their lower levels of interest in objects in general (Kasari and Freeman, 2001). The implication for pragmatic intervention is that attention to cognitive and linguistic limitations may be not be sufficient – broader personality-motivational factors may need to be targeted as well.

Several researchers have also looked to nonverbally expressed interpersonal goals for the origins of the especially serious problems in receptive and especially expressive language that ultimately characterize the vast majority of individuals with Down syndrome (Chapman and Hesketh, 2000). Motivating this research is the *continuity hypothesis* proposed within work on typical development, which includes the claim that nonverbal communicative achievements provide a necessary foundation for later, linguistic, acquisitions (for example, Bates and Thal, 1991). Studies of children with Down syndrome have been consistent with the continuity hypothesis in demonstrating a positive relationship between measures of nonverbal communication and later language skills. In particular, both Mundy and his colleagues (Mundy et al., 1988, 1995) and Smith and Von Tetzchner (1986) found that after statistically controlling initial language level, the rate of nonverbal requests for objects predicted concurrent and subsequent expressive language, as assessed by the Reynell Developmental Language Scales (1977). Elsewhere (Abbeduto and Hesketh, 1997) we have suggested that this relationship may reflect the fact that nonverbal requesting might facilitate lexical learning by providing an opportunity for adult care providers to supply object labels when the child with Down syndrome is most interested in the object. The implication for intervention is that language forms may not be learnable independent of the interpersonal goals, or speech acts, that typically motivate their use. In some cases, this may necessitate targeting absent pragmatic skills before the relevant linguistic forms.

Children with Down syndrome are substantially delayed in making the transition from nonverbal communication into 'true' language (Berglund, 2001). Interestingly, the serious deficits in the manner of non-verbal commenting and the frequency of nonverbal requesting observed for children with Down syndrome have not been reported by researchers studying the speech acts expressed linguistically by children with Down syndrome (Abbeduto and Hesketh, 1997). In fact, this latter research has generally found that children with Down syndrome use language to express the same speech acts and at the same relative rates as do younger typically developing children at similar levels of linguistic or cognitive development (Coggins, Carpenter and Owings, 1983). So, for example, preschoolers with Down syndrome and expressive language-matched typically developing toddlers have been found to make the greatest use of the speech act of 'answering' when interacting with their mothers (Owens and MacDonald, 1982). Such results suggest that at least during the early stages of language learning, children with Down syndrome view language as a vehicle for achieving the same interpersonal goals as do typically developing children. However, this research has involved only analyses of parent–child interaction, which leaves open the question of how extensively the language use of the children with Down syndrome who were studied has been supported or shaped by parents. It is possible that these children might not look as skilled if observed interacting with peers, who will be less adept at structuring the interaction to achieve the optimal performance from the child with Down syndrome (Rosenberg and Abbeduto, 1993).

Researchers interested in mental retardation and Down syndrome have focused not only on language expression but also on comprehension; that is, the ways in which affected individuals recognize the linguistically expressed speech acts of other people. In this research, individuals with mental retardation, regardless of etiology, have been found to be delayed (relative to age-matched typically developing peers) in their comprehension (Rosenberg and Abbeduto, 1993). This is not surprising because comprehension requires not only a familiarity with the words and combinatorial rules of a language, but also an ability to integrate that information with a variety of sources of contextual information. This is the case because any language form can be used to perform different interpersonal goals in different contexts and the same goal can be accomplished by uttering many different forms (Levinson, 1983). In the context of naturally occurring play with parents, children with Down syndrome respond appropriately to parental requests for actions (for example, 'can you put the piece in the puzzle?') as often as would be expected for their levels of nonverbal cognitive functioning (Leifer and Lewis, 1984). This may reflect an ability to use contextual information to make inferences about speech acts – an ability that is known to depend heavily on a variety of cognitive skills (Abbeduto and Rosenberg, 1992). Again, however, it is difficult to generalize beyond parent-child interactions. It may be that, in less familiar circumstances or with less skilled partners, the level of comprehension demonstrated by individuals with Down syndrome may be less well developed than suggested by studies to date. It is interesting to note that although tied closely to cognitive development, the level of understanding of speech acts demonstrated by individuals with Down syndrome (Leifer and Lewis, 1984) as well as by individuals with mental retardation of various other etiologies (Abbeduto, Davies and Furman, 1988) often exceeds their maturity in mastery of language forms and contents, which is consistent with a variety of claims about the dissociability of various 'components' of language (for example, Rondal, 1995; but see Abbeduto et al., 2001). Such findings suggest that not all 'gaps' in an individual's linguistic system may have consequences for everyday communication. The implication for intervention is that the emphasis should be on maximizing pragmatic skill, which may sometimes require training the individual in the use of forms already in his or her repertoire rather than always introducing new language forms.

There is much that we do not know about the speech act expression and comprehension of individuals with Down syndrome. We know little about development in this domain beyond the preschool years. This is unfortunate because there is some evidence (for example, Abbeduto and Rosenberg, 1980) that adults with mental retardation of other etiologies become quite skilled in this domain. Determining whether this same favourable outcome characterizes Down syndrome would help to establish the need for, and optimal timing of, intervention in this area. We also lack data on individual differences in speech act expression and comprehension among individuals with Down syndrome. Such data, along with an understanding of the causes of those differences, are essential for the development of effective programme of assessment and intervention.

Establishing the referents of the talk

It is critical for successful communication of one's interpersonal goals that the participants understand to which entities or events each and every utterance refers. Being unclear as to who *he* and *it* are in the utterance *he did it* makes the utterance all but vacuous. Similarly, the utterance *could I have that toy?* uttered with only a vague gesture in the direction of a closet full of toys will not get the speaker the object he or she desires. Making clear the referents of one's talk when in the role of speaker and using all the linguistic and situational information at hand to identify the partner's referents when in the role of listener are thus foundational skills for participation in linguistic interactions (Abbeduto and Hesketh, 1997). In pragmatics, the study of these skills falls within the topic of *referential communication.*

There has been ample documentation that persons with mental retardation, whatever the etiology, are especially challenged when it comes to producing messages that make their intended referents clear to others (Rosenberg and Abbeduto, 1993). Indeed, children, adolescents, and adults with mental retardation have been found to perform less well in this area than would be expected from their levels of nonlinguistic cognitive functioning (Abbeduto, Weissman and Short-Meyerson, 1999). Not surprisingly, therefore, recent studies have suggested that individuals with Down syndrome also have great difficulty in establishing the referents of their talk when in the role of speaker. In an examination of narrative production, for example, Boudreau and Chapman (2000) found that 12 to 26-year-olds with Down syndrome were less likely to correctly introduce referents into their stories than were cognitively matched typically developing 2 to 8-year-olds. In fact, the referent introductions of these adolescents and young adults with Down syndrome were more similar to those of typically developing children with equivalent expressive language skills.

Are the referential difficulties of individuals with Down syndrome different in either degree or kind from the difficulties displayed by individuals with mental retardation of other etiologies? Unfortunately, there are few data addressing this question. There is evidence demonstrating that the referential problems of individuals with Down syndrome may be less severe than are those of adults with autism (Loveland, Tunali, McEvoy and Kelly, 1989). However, data from Abbeduto and his colleagues (Abbeduto, 2001) suggest that there are commonalities as well as differences across syndromes in this domain. They used a non-face-to-face task in which the participant needed to talk to an adult listener about a set of novel shapes. The use of novel shapes ensured that the participant had no ready labels for the shape but instead needed to collaborate with the listener to create a system of shared reference that worked for them both. Moreover, each shape recurred several times across trials, which enabled examination of the extent to which the participant's talk about each shaped changed as the system of reference and the knowledge shared with the listener evolved. In addition to including adolescents and young adults with Down syndrome as participants, Abbeduto (2001) included adolescents and young adults with fragile X syndrome, an X-linked inherited disorder often leading to mental retardation (Abbeduto and Hagerman, 1997).

Abbeduto and colleagues found that both the participants with Down syndrome and those with fragile X syndrome were less able to create *unique mappings* between their descriptions and the shapes than were typically developing 3- to 6-year-olds matched to them in terms of nonverbal cognitive ability. By a unique mapping, Abbeduto and colleagues (2001) meant instances in which a participant used a particular description for only one shape rather than extending it to multiple shapes; for example, saying something like 'the ice cream cone' for one and only one of the shapes they needed to talk about over trials. Unique mappings would contrast with indiscriminate mappings, which would make the listener's task of referent identification far more difficult. Suppose, for example, 'the ice cream cone' might refer to more than one of the shapes. How would the listener know which shape was being talked about for sure on any given trial if the participant had previously used it for more than one shape?

It was also found by Abbeduto and colleagues (2001) that the participants with Down syndrome did more poorly than either the participants with fragile X syndrome or the typically developing children in providing a scaffolding for their listener through the use of what were called *referential frames*. Examples of the use of referential frames would be 'it's kind of an ice cream cone' (rather than simply 'it's an ice cream cone') or 'it looks like a house' (rather than simply 'it's a house'). Referential frames provide additional guidance for the listener by pointing out that the noun phrase describes a similarity between the shape and a real object rather than 'being' that object. It was found that the participants with Down syndrome, as a group, were less likely to use referential frames than was either of the other two groups. Moreover, this seemed to be a manifestation of the serious expressive language limitations that many individuals with Down syndrome display (Chapman and Hesketh, 2000). This is suggested by the finding that scores on standardized measures of language ability, especially expressive language ability, were highly predictive of the use of referential frames by the participants.

These results suggest that many aspects of referential communication are especially problematic for individuals with Down syndrome, with some problems perhaps being syndrome specific and others being common not only to Down syndrome but also to fragile X syndrome. Importantly, Abbeduto et al. also identified areas of strength in the performance of the participants with Down syndrome. In particular, as a group, they were as adept as were the typically developing comparison children at changing their referential talk over repeated occurrences of a particular shape, as the system of reference and the knowledge shared with the listener evolved. For example, they took less time to complete their referential exchanges and were more likely to use definite rather than indefinite articles on later trials compared to earlier trials, and did not differ from the typically developing children in this regard. These results show the value of comparing the pragmatic performance of individuals with Down syndrome to that of other well-defined syndromes – it provides the foundation for assessments and interventions that are tailored to the specific profile of strengths and weaknesses that define Down syndrome.

There remains much that we do not know about this fundamental aspect of pragmatics in individuals with Down syndrome. It is not known, for example, how skilled individuals with Down syndrome are in working to identify the referents of the talk heard when in the role of listener. The listener must do more than simply process the linguistic form of the speaker's message. The listener must, for example, also integrate the information in the speaker's utterance with information gleaned from the discourse to that point, the physical context, and the speaker's nonverbal behaviour (Anderson, Clark and Mullin, 1994). There also is a need for data on the referential communication of individuals with Down syndrome in both the speaker and listener role across a wider range of face-to-face and non-face-to-face tasks reflective of the many types of social interactions in which people with Down syndrome participate on a daily basis.

Topic as the context for talk

A linguistic interaction is more than just a haphazard collection of requests, comments, answers, and the like. Instead, an interaction has an organization. This organization emerges out of the activities and events in which the participants in the talk are engaged (Schegloff, 1990). For example, the talk of two children playing 'dress up' is shaped by that activity such that what is said moves the play forward toward some desired end state, and the sequence of the talk (and the interpersonal goals underlying it) is determined by, and makes sense only within, the context of that play. In the case of two adults who are catching up on the comings and goings in their neighbourhood, the sequencing of their talk is determined by, and interpretable only within, the activity of gossiping. It is useful to think of these activities that organize talk as the *topic* of that talk. Collaborating with one's discourse partner to ensure that the topic moves forward is a demanding pragmatic task. It requires that we design what we say so that it is sensible, or 'fits,' in light of what has already been said (Abbeduto and Short-Meyerson, 2002). It also requires creating an opportunity for one's partners to build on one's own contribution (Ninio and Snow, 1996). Contributing to the topic in this way also places heavy demands on cognitive ability because it requires tracking the progression of the topic at hand, as well as knowledge of the objects and events that define the topic (Short-Meyerson and Abbeduto, 1997). It also requires knowledge of the linguistic forms that are conventionally used to mark the introduction of new topics and the ending of current topics (Brinton and Fujiki, 1989).

It might be supposed that the broad range of skills involved in 'controlling' the topic would make this a particularly challenging aspect of pragmatics for individuals with mental retardation, including those with Down syndrome. However, there have been few studies of topic control that have focused on individuals with Down syndrome and most, whether focused on Down syndrome or more broadly on mental retardation, have typically relied on measures (for example, topic length) that may not accurately reflect topic quality (Abbeduto and Hesketh, 1997). In one of the few studies involving children with Down syndrome, Tannock (1988) found that young children with Down syndrome were less likely to introduce new topics in conversations with their mothers than were typically developing children matched to them on level of cognitive and linguistic ability. It is difficult to know, however, whether this reflects a lack of topic skills on the part of children with Down syndrome or a lack of opportunity to introduce topics as a result of high maternal control of the conversation (Abbeduto and Hesketh, 1997). Tannock also found that these children with Down syndrome and their mothers maintained their topics for about as long as did the matched typically developing children and their mothers. Again, however, we do not know the extent to which this reflects the skills of the children with Down syndrome or the skills of their mothers. Moreover, it is not clear that topic length is actually a good measure of topic quality (Rosenberg and Abbeduto, 1993). Indeed, there may be instances in which staying on topic reflects perseveration, or a repetition of the topic without progress toward closure or the addition of new information (Pavetto, 2001).

Clearly, much more attention needs to be devoted to learning about the topic skills of individuals with Down syndrome so that we can decide if interventions are needed and if so, what form they should take and how they should be evaluated. A recent study by Berglund (2001) suggests that such attention is warranted. In particular, Berglund used parent report to investigate several dimensions of language development in a large sample of Swedish-speaking children with Down syndrome. Included were questions about the children's talk about different types of topics, such as past/future events, absent objects/persons, and expression of ownership. Berglund found, among other things, that many children were reported to have not talked about any of the topics. This suggests that further work on topic might do well to focus on the nature of the events that engender (or fail to engender) talk in individuals with Down syndrome. Such work will need to evaluate the ways in which the world knowledge of individuals with Down syndrome and the events in which their talk is embedded impact their contributions to the topic (Short-Meyerson and Abbeduto, 1997). Hopefully, future research on topic will also include comparison with other etiologies so that we can learn about the syndrome specificity of any topic problems identified.

Evaluating self- and other-understanding of language

Because the general goal of any linguistic interaction is to achieve some semblance of a meeting of the minds, it is important that the participants in the interaction monitor the extent to which this occurs. If this is not done, there is little chance that either the mutual or the idiosyncratic interpersonal goals of the participants will be achieved. In the role of speaker, the participants must engage in behaviours to ensure that their utterances have been understood in the way intended, behaviours which Clark (1996) has referred to as *grounding*. These behaviours include monitoring the listener's reactions to utterances (for example, looking for signs of confusion, such as a puzzled facial expression) and if necessary actively soliciting information about his or her understanding (for example, 'know what I mean?'). Grounding also involves responding to explicit signals of non-comprehension (for example, 'which one?') from the listener by clarifying problematic points and messages. Listeners also participate in this grounding process (Clark, 1996) by, among other things, acknowledging verbally (for example, 'OK') or nonverbally (for example, by nodding in agreement) the speaker's utterance and by formulating signals of non-comprehension that specify the nature of the problems to be corrected (for example, 'there are two like that').

Considerable research has been conducted into the ways in which persons with mental retardation participate in the grounding process both as listeners and speakers (Abbeduto and Hesketh, 1997; Abbeduto and Short-Meyerson, 2002). Little of this research, however, has focused specifically on individuals with Down syndrome. In fact, there have been no studies of grounding from the perspective of listeners with Down syndrome. Thus, we do not know how skilled individuals with Down syndrome are at monitoring their comprehension and signaling in an informative manner when they fail to understand. This is unfortunate because there is considerable evidence that this is an area of delay, perhaps even greater than expected for mental age delay, for persons with mental retardation in general (Abbeduto, Davies, Solesby and Furman, 1991; Abbeduto, Short-Meyerson, Benson and Dolish, 1997). Moreover, it is an area in which interventions have been developed and shown to be successful for children with mental retardation (Ezell and Goldstein, 1991).

There has been research, however, on the extent to which individuals with Down syndrome, as speakers, deal effectively with signals of non-comprehension from others. Coggins and Stoel-Gammon (1982) and Scherer and Owings (1984) examined the responses of preschoolers with Down syndrome to non-comprehension signals from adults in a variety of naturally occurring daily activities, from mealtimes to free play. These investigators found that the children responded to nearly all of the adult signals, albeit in ways that were less mature than expected for their chronological ages. The lack of appropriate comparison groups, however, makes it difficult to know whether the responses of the children with Down syndrome were appropriate for their developmental levels. Until such data are collected, the need for interventions targeting this aspect of pragmatics is unclear.

Clearly, there is much to be learned about the extent and effectiveness of the grounding behaviours of individuals with Down syndrome. An area that has received no attention, either in studies of Down syndrome or individuals with mental retardation more generally, is the 'positive' side of grounding; that is, the extent to which, and how, these individuals signal when they *do* understand what others have said or whether, and how, they solicit such positive feedback from others.

Enhancing pragmatic abilities

Despite the large literature on language interventions with individuals having mental retardation, interventions specifically targeting pragmatic deficits rather than the acquisition of language forms have been surprisingly rare (Rosenberg and Abbeduto, 1993). Research directed at evaluating pragmatic interventions for individuals with Down syndrome or comparing the effectiveness of an intervention across Down syndrome and other etiological groups has been even less frequent. Moreover, many interventions have not been guided by either a model of mature pragmatic performance or have not been well informed about pragmatic development in individuals with Down syndrome or typically developing children. Unfortunately, this has often led to interventions that, should they achieve their intended targets, are unlikely to result in any noticeable improvement in the real-life social interactions of the individuals treated (Rosenberg and Abbeduto, 1993).

Nevertheless, there is reason to be optimistic. There is empirical evidence that individuals with Down syndrome and other forms of cognitive disabilities can improve their pragmatic language or social skills through participation in intervention programmes. These interventions have embodied one of two approaches:

- A naturalistic approach, such as milieu or responsive integrative teaching, which typically has as its goal the acquisition of new language forms and the ability to use those forms in pragmatically appropriate ways (MacDonald, 1989; Warren, Yoder, Gazdag, Kim and Jones 1993; Yoder and Warren, 1998; Warren and Yoder, 1998); and
- Behavioural techniques used to increase the frequency of use of specific, rather narrowly defined, pragmatic skills.

Naturalistic interventions are implemented within the context of the child's everyday environments and are responsive to, and controlled by, the child's spontaneously occurring behaviour. Behavioural interventions are typically conducted within more structured environments and are didactic in nature, involving a high degree of adult control.

Naturalistic approaches

There are several principles that underlie the naturalistic approaches. First, they require the creation of an environment that provides opportunities to communicate by fostering the child's desire to address specific interpersonal goals. For example, Warren and Yoder (1998) suggest that the child's environment should contain materials that are of interest to the child and, ideally, should be placed in a position where an adult's assistance is necessary to reach them, thereby prompting the child's need to communicate with the adult about the goal. Second, the approaches assume that children are more interactive and attentive when they choose the object or activity instead of being directed towards the choices of others (MacDonald, 1989). This nondirective style involves following the child's lead by providing him or her with a more developmentally advanced or pragmatically effective linguistic (or nonlinguistic) means of achieving the desired interpersonal goal he or she has just attempted to address. Third, it has been assumed that social routines (rituals or activities that are highly repetitive and familiar to the child) are the context in which children typically learn language, and thus routines are thought to be highly effective in facilitating new pragmatic achievements (Warren, 1991; Warren and Yoder, 1998; Yoder and Davies, 1992a; Yoder and Davies, 1992b).

The most well-studied naturalistic approach is the *milieu approach*. Milieu interventions are typically conducted in a child's school or home and they involve responding to naturally occurring teaching opportunities created by the child's attempts at communication. They also involve selecting behavioural targets according to well-established typical sequences of development. For example, the child might reach and vocalize to signal a desire for an out-of-reach toy. If the intervention plan includes the increased use of single-word requests, the adult might respond, not by getting the toy, but by naming it (for example, 'ball') followed by a prompt for the child to do the same (for example, 'say, "ball"'). This approach can be implemented by teachers, clinicians or other professionals who focus directly on altering the pragmatic behaviours of the targeted child (Warren, 1991). Alternatively, the approach can be designed to alter the behaviour of the adults who regularly interact with the targeted child during the normal course of his or her day (for example, the child's parents). In this latter case, the approach involves teaching the adults how to interact with, and respond to, the child's attempts at communication (Warren, 1991). In both instantiations of the approach, there are empirical demonstrations of its effectiveness.

In a study by Warren et al. (1993), the effectiveness of a milieu approach teaching a single 20-month-old prelinguistic boy with Down syndrome was investigated. The intervention was designed to increase the frequency of three nonverbally expressed interpersonal goals, or 'speech' acts: requesting, commenting and vocal imitation. It was found that the boy exhibited an increase in the frequency of requests, comments, and vocal imitations after the intervention. In a second study involving four children with various kinds of developmental disabilities, the results indicated that the milieu teaching approach was effective in increasing the children's rates of the three target behaviours, as well as in facilitating generalization across contexts and encouraging changes in the classroom teachers' interaction with the children. In a larger study of 58 children with developmental disabilities, Warren and colleagues demonstrated that prelinguistic milieu teaching was effective in improving intentional communication, particularly in children of mothers who were responsive before treatment. Together these studies by Warren and his colleagues suggest that prelinguistic milieu teaching is an effective method of increasing intentional communication, especially when it is consistent with the interactional style and history of the adults implementing it.

Behavioural approaches

Although studies have examined the effectiveness of behavioural techniques in improving pragmatic ability, a number of these studies are case studies or involve a very small number of participants. In a study of six children with mental retardation of varying etiology, Halle, Marshall and Spradlin (1979) utilized a 15-second delay following a child's 'arrival' in a context in which the adult's assistance was required to increase the number of verbal requests during meals. They reported that three of the children increased the number of verbal requests with only the delay, and two of the remaining three showed improvement when modelling of the desired request was combined with the delay. Using a similar delay procedure, Halle, Baer and Spradlin (1981) reported generalization of treatment effects to novel settings. Gobbi, Cipani, Hudson and Lapenta-Neudeck (1986) used a 30-second delay combined with prompts and models to increase spontaneous requests in two children with developmental disabilities. This behaviour was maintained in a one-month follow-up. McCook, Cipani, Madigan and LaCampagne (1988) reported similar results with two adults with mental retardation. Despite the effectiveness of these interventions, their application to heterogeneous groups of participants who are sometimes poorly described as regards etiology, makes it impossible to know the extent to which the interventions would be effective in improving the requesting and other speech act behaviour of individuals with Down syndrome.

A few studies have been conducted to examine the effectiveness of interventions focused on topic initiation and maintenance (Downing, 1987; Haring, Roger, Lee, Breen and Gaylord-Ross, 1986). For example, Downing (1987) attempted to teach three adolescents with mental retardation how to initiate and maintain a conversation. Downing reported an increase in both behaviours but there was minimal generalization of the treatment effects to unfamiliar adults. Other studies have examined the effectiveness of self-monitoring to improve topic skills (Matson and Adkins, 1980; Schloss and Wood, 1990). Again, however, the relative efficacy of these interventions for individuals with Down syndrome compared to those whose mental retardation of other origins remains to be determined.

In summary, these studies support the effectiveness of treatment programs to improve the pragmatic abilities of children and adults with cognitive disabilities. Few of these studies, however, have included individuals with Down syndrome or examined the effectiveness of the intervention for them alone. Clearly, more studies of interventions that involve etiological comparisons involving Down syndrome are needed. Moreover, existing data on pragmatic interventions have been obtained from a small number of case studies or small sample studies. Future research should include experimental designs utilizing large sample sizes. There also are many important pragmatic skills that have been largely ignored in intervention work, including comprehension of speech acts, establishing referents, and evaluation of self- and other-understanding of language in the context of social interaction. Finally, evaluation of treatment effects is also an important research goal.

References

Abbeduto L (2001) Syndrome Differences in Language and Communication: A Comparison of Down Syndrome and Fragile X Syndrome. Annual meeting of the Symposium for Research on Child Language Disorders, Madison Wis, June.

Abbeduto L, Benson G (1992) Speech act development in nondisabled children and individuals with mental retardation. In R Chapman (ed.) Processes in Language Acquisition and Disorders. Chicago: Mosby-Yearbook, pp. 257–78.

Abbeduto L, Davies B, Furman L (1988) The development of speech act comprehension in mentally retarded individuals and nonretarded children. Child Development 59: 1460–72.

Abbeduto L, Davies B, Solesby S, Furman L (1991) Identifying the referents of spoken messages: the use of context and clarification requests by children with and without mental retardation. American Journal on Mental Retardation 95: 551–62.

Abbeduto L, Evans J, Dolan T (2001) Theoretical perspectives on language and communication problems in mental retardation and developmental disabilities. Mental Retardation and Developmental Disabilities Research Reviews 7: 45–55.

Abbeduto L, Hagerman R (1997) Language and communication in fragile X syndrome. Mental Retardation and Developmental Disabilities Research Reviews 3: 313–22.

Abbeduto L, Hesketh LJ (1997) Pragmatic development in individuals with mental retardation: learning to use language in social interactions. Mental Retardation and Developmental Disabilities Research Reviews 3: 323–33.

Abbeduto L, Pavetto M, Kesin E, Weissman MD, Karadottir S, O'Brien A, Cawthon S (in press) The Language and Cognitive Profile of Down Syndrome: Evidence from a Comparison with Fragile X Syndrome. Down Syndrome Research and Practice.

Abbeduto L, Rosenberg S (1980) The communicative competence of mildly retarded adults. Applied Psycholinguistics 1: 405–26.

Abbeduto L, Rosenberg S (1992) The development of linguistic communication in persons with mental retardation. In S Warren, J Reichle (eds) Causes and effects in communication and language intervention. Baltimore Md: Brookes, pp. 331–59.

Abbeduto L, Short-Meyerson K (in press) Linguistic influences on social interaction. In H Goldstein, L Kaczmarek, KM English (eds) Promoting Social Communication in Children and Youth with Developmental Disabilities. Baltimore: Brookes.

Abbeduto L, Short-Meyerson K, Benson G, Dolish J (1997) Signaling of noncomprehension by children and adolescents with mental retardation: effects of problem type and speaker identity. Journal of Speech, Language, and Hearing Research 40: 20–32.

Abbeduto L, Short-Meyerson K, Benson G, Dolish J, Weissman M (1998) Understanding referential expressions: use of common ground by children and adolescents with mental retardation. Journal of Speech, Language, and Hearing Research 41: 348–62.

Abbeduto L, Weissman MD, Short-Meyerson K (1999) Parental scaffolding of the discourse of children and adolescents with mental retardation: the case of referential expressions. Journal of Intellectual Disability Research 43: 540–57.

Anderson AH, Clark A, Mullin J (1994) Interactive communication between children: learning how to make language work in dialogue. Journal of Child Language 21: 439–64.

Bates E, Thal D (1991) Associations and dissociations in language development. In J Miller (ed.) Research on Child Language Disorders: A Decade of Progress. Austin, Tex: Peo-ED, pp. 145–68.

Berglund EEMJI (2001) Parental reports of spoken language skills in children with Down syndrome. Journal of Speech, Language and Hearing Research 44: 179–91.

Boudreau DM, Chapman RS (2000) The relationship between event representation and linguistic skill in narratives of children and adolescents with Down syndrome. Journal of Speech, Language and Hearing Research 43: 1146–59.

Brinton B, Fujiki M (1989) Conversational Management with Language-Impaired Children: Pragmatic assessment and intervention. Gaithersburg Md: Aspen.

Chapman RS, Hesketh LJ (2000) The behavioural phenotype of individuals with Down syndrome. Mental Retardation and Developmental Disabilities Research Reviews 6: 84–95.

Clark HH (1996) Using Language. New York: Cambridge University Press.

Coggins TE, Carpenter RL, Owings NO (1983) Examining early intentional communication in Down's syndrome and nonretarded children. British Journal of Disorders of Communication 18: 98–106.

Coggins TE, Stoel-Gammon C (1982) Clarification strategies used by four Down's syndrome children for maintaining normal conversational interaction. Education and Training of the Mentally Retarded 17: 65–7.

Downing J (1987) Conversational skills training: teaching adolescents with mental retardation to be verbally assertive. Mental Retardation 25: 147–55.

Ezell HK, Goldstein H (1991) Observational learning of comprehension monitoring skills in children who exhibit mental retardation. Journal of Speech and Hearing Research 34: 141–54.

Fabbretti D, Pizzuto E, Vicari S, Volterra V (1997) A story description task in children with Down's syndrome: lexical and morphosyntactic abilities. Journal of Intellectual Disability Research 41: 165–79.

Gobbi L, Cipani E, Hudson C, Lapenta-Neudeck R (1986) Developing spontaneous requesting among children with severe mental retardation. Mental Retardation 24: 357–63.

Graesser AC, Millis KK, Zwaan RA (1997) Discourse comprehension. In JT Spence, JM Darley, DJ Foss (eds) Annual Review of Psychology. Palo Alto Calif: The Annual Reviews Inc, pp. 163–89.

Greenwald CA, Leonard LB (1979) Communicative and sensorimotor development of Down's syndrome children. American Journal on Mental Deficiency 84: 296–303.

Halle J, Baer D, Spradlin J (1981) Teachers' generalized use of delay as a stimulus control procedure to increase language use in handicapped children. Journal of Applied Behaviour Analysis 14: 389–409.

Halle J, Marshall A, Spradlin J (1979) Time delay: a technique to increase language use and facilitate generalization in retarded children. Journal of Applied Behaviour Analysis 12: 431–9.

Haring T, Roger B, Lee M, Breen C, Gaylord-Ross R (1986) Teaching social language to moderately handicapped students. American Journal on Mental Retardation 19: 159–71.

Kasari C, Freeman SFN (2001) Task-related social behaviour in children with Down syndrome. American Journal on Mental Retardation 106: 253–64.

Leifer JS, Lewis M (1984) Acquisition of conversational response skills by young Down syndrome and nonretarded young children. American Journal of Mental Deficiency 88: 610–18.

Levinson SC (1983) Pragmatics. Cambridge: Cambridge University Press.

Loveland KA, Tunali B, McEvoy RE, Loveland K, Kelley ML (1989) Referential communication and response adequacy in autism and Down's syndrome. Applied Psycholinguistics 10: 301–13.

Marcell MM, Weeks SL (1988) Short-term memory difficulties and Down's syndrome. Journal of Mental Deficiency Research 32: 153–62.

MacDonald J (1989) Becoming Partners with Children: From Play to Conversation. San Antonio: Special Press Inc.

McCook B, Cipani E, Madigan K, LaCampagne J (1988) Developing requesting behaviour: acquisition, fluency, and generality. Mental Retardation 26: 137–43.

Matson JL, Adkins J (1980) A self-instructional social skills training program for mentally retarded persons. Mental Retardation 18: 245–8.

Mundy P, Signamn M, Kasari C, Yirmia N (1988) Nonverbal communication skills in Down syndrome children. Child Development 59: 235–49.

Mundy P, Kasari C, Sigman M, Ruskin E (1995). Nonverbal communication and early language acquisition in children with Down syndrome and normally developing children. Journal of Speech and Hearing Research 38: 157–67.

Ninio A, Snow CE (1996) Pragmatic Development. Boulder Colo: Westview Press.

Owens RE Jr, MacDonald JD (1982) Communicative uses of the early speech of nondelayed and Down syndrome children. American Journal of Mental Deficiency 86: 503–10.

Pavetto MM (2001) Gender differences in repetitive language among adolescents with fragile X syndrome. Unpublished master's thesis, University of Wisconsin-Madison, Madison Wis.

Piaget J (1952) The Origins of Intelligence in Children (translated M.Cook, Trans.). New York: International Universities Press.

Rondal JA (1995) Exceptional Language Development in Down Syndrome: Implications for the Cognition-Language Relationship. Cambridge: Cambridge University Press.

Rosenberg S, Abbeduto L (1993). Language and Communication in Mental Retardation: Development, Processes, and Intervention. Hillsdale NJ: Erlbaum.

Schegloff EA (1990) On the organization of sequences as a source of 'coherence' in talk-in-interaction. In B Dorval (ed.) Conversational Organization and its Development. Norwood NJ: Ablex, pp. 51–77.

Scherer NJ, Owings NO (1984) Learning to be contingent: retarded children's responses to their mothers' requests. Language and Speech 27: 255–67.

Schloss PJ, Wood CE (1990) Effect of self-monitoring on maintenance and generalization of conversational skills of persons with mental retardation. Mental Retardation 28: 105–13.

Short-Meyerson K, Abbeduto L (1997) Preschoolers' communication during scripted interaction. Journal of Child Language 24: 469–93.

Smith L, Von Tetzchner S (1986) Communicative, sensorimotor, and language skills of young children with Down syndrome. American Journal on Mental Deficiency 91: 57–66.

Tannock R (1988) Mother directiveness in their interactions with their children with and without Down syndrome. American Journal on Mental Retardation 93: 154–65.

Warren S (1991) Enhancing communication and language development with milieu teaching procedures. In E Cipani (ed.) A Guide for Developing Language Competence in Preschool Children with Severe and Moderate Handicaps. Springfield Ill: Charles C Thomas, pp. 68–93.

Warren S, Yoder P (1998) Facilitating the transition from preintentional to intentional communication. In A Wetherby, S Warren, J Reichle (eds) Transitions in Prelinguistic Communication. Baltimore: Paul H Brookes, pp. 365–84.

Warren S, Yoder P, Gazdag GE, Kim K, Jones HA (1993) Facilitating prelinguistic communication skills in young children with developmental delay. Journal of Speech and Hearing Research 36(1): 83–97.

Yoder PJ, Davies B (1992a) Do children with developmental delays use more frequent and diverse language in verbal routines? American Journal on Mental Retardation 97(2): 197–208.

Yoder PJ, Davies B (1992b) Greater intelligibility in verbal routines with young children with developmental delays. Applied Psycholinguistics 13(1): 77–91.

Yoder PJ, Warren SF (1998) Maternal responsivity predicts the prelinguistic communication intervention that facilitates generalized intentional communication. Journal of Speech, Language, and Hearing Research 41(5): 1207–19.

Acknowledgement

Preparation of this manuscript was supported by grants R01 HD23546, P30 HD03352, and T32 HD07489, all from the National Institutes of Health.

Chapter 8
Augmentative communication

GAYE POWELL, JOHN CLIBBENS

Over the past quarter of a century therapeutic approaches for individuals who are vulnerable in terms of communication and language development, particularly those at risk of developing little or no intelligible speech, have increasingly included augmentative and alternative modes of communication (AAC) (Von Tetzchner and Jensen, 1996; Beukelman and Mirenda, 1998). For those with Down syndrome whose speech and language development is generally delayed relative to cognitive, social and motor skills AAC has been considered to offer a positive contribution to communication development. Augmentative and alternative communication in the form of keyword manual signing has been the most frequently researched modality in relation to early language development (LeProvost, 1983; Miller, 1992; Launonen, 1996, 1998) and the communication of adults in this client group (Grove and Walker, 1990; Powell and Clibbens, 1994). However, more technical communication aids and computers are now increasingly included for assistive purposes to enhance and extend communication abilities either on a temporary or permanent basis depending upon current need (Murray-Branch and Gamradt, 1999).

Terminology

Although the term 'AAC' was initially applied to a range of graphic symbol systems used to enable communication in individuals with cerebral palsy and other motor difficulties (Kates and McNaughton, 1975; see Zangari, Lloyd and Vicker, 1994 and Beukelman and Mirenda, 1998 for overviews and historical developments), it now encompasses an array of modalities that may be used in combination with, or in the absence of, speech. This includes the use of manual/gestural keyword signs that have been adapted from the indigenous sign language of the country, such as Makaton

(Walker, 1976), visual/pictographic symbols that vary in their level of complexity (Bliss, 1965; Walker, Parsons, Cousins, Carpenter and Park, 1985), tangible symbols and representational and real objects (Grove and Walker, 1990; Schweigert and Rowland, 1998; see Von Tetzchner and Jensen, 1996 for a review of European perspectives). The terms bimodal and multimodal have also evolved to reflect the relationships across, and between, modalities where speech is not the primary, or only, means of accessing or producing language (Smith and Grove, in press). Lonke, van der Beken and Lloyd, 1998 (cited in Smith and Grove, in press) further extend this to distinguish between 'parallel multimodality' where speech is accompanied by gesture or sign, and 'recoded multimodality' where there is re-formulation from one mode to another. In the latter communication contexts speech tends to be the main input mode whilst output (by the communicatively impaired partner) is by a distinctly different mode such as a graphic symbol and does not occur simultaneously with speech.

Communication development in Down syndrome

There are exceptions (Rondal, 1995) but anecdotal and empirical evidence indicates that individuals with Down syndrome generally present with a delayed pattern of speech and language development at all stages (Fowler, 1990; Buckley, 1993; Jenkins, 1993; Fowler, Gelman and Gleitman, 1994; Lynch et al, 1995; Cobo-Lewis, Kimbrough Oller, Lynch, and Levine, 1996; Franco and Wishart, 1996; Remington and Clarke, 1996; Rondal, 1996; Stoel-Gammon, 1997). This is known to be associated with a range of neurological anomalies (Schmidt-Sidor, Wisniewski, Shepard, and Sersen, 1990) but no single cause has yet been identified (Chapman, 1997; see Rondal, Perera, Nadel, and Comblain, 1996 for a review). However, given the profile of frequently associated difficulties that may constrain language acquisition and use (Buckley, 1993), including intermittent hearing loss and poor oro-motor skills, AAC would appear to be a favourable addition to the range of therapeutic options available (see Remington and Clarke 1996 for an earlier consideration of AAC and Down syndrome). Despite a number of studies providing evidence to the contrary (Foreman and Crews, 1998; LeProvost, 1993; Powell and Clibbens, 1994; Sisson and Barrett, 1984; see Parsons and Wills, 1992 and Powell, 1999 for a review) parental fears still exist that the use of AAC may have a negative effect upon speech and language development (Parsons and Wills, 1992), in particular that:

- AAC may prevent the development of verbal language
- introducing AAC is an indication that speech is being abandoned as a potential means of expression and focus for therapy
- using AAC will be an additional stigma in a predominantly speaking world

- AAC, particularly manual signs, will be difficult for the child and family to learn (Foreman and Crews, 1998).

These points will be revisited later as whilst the first two may be countered by research findings, it is possible that the last two continue to constrain individuals from attaining their language potential and require more careful consideration if programmes of intervention are to be effective.

Multimodality

On the surface, introducing 'new' additional/alternative modes of communication to young children could be perceived as potentially confusing. However, research has shown that typically developing infants integrate a number of modalities to communicate prior to the development of speech as the primary linguistic mode. These include gesture, body movements, facial expression and vocalizations (Capirci, Iverson, Pizzuto, and Volterra, 1996; Grove, 1997; Smith, 1997; Roy and Panayi, 1997). Over time, the strength and relevance of the different modes to the communication context changes as children become more proficient within each mode (intramodal development cf Smith, 1997) and learn to manipulate them in relation to one another (intermodal development, cf Smith, 1997). Within these modalities two distinct categories of gesture are described: 'deictic' and 'representation' (Capirci, Iverson, Pizzuto, and Volterra, 1996). Deictic gestures emerge during the prelinguistic period and are used to request, declare, and draw attention, be it joint or otherwise, to an object or location in the given physical context. Such gestures are not representational or symbolic but may gain such status in the interpretation of intention assigned by the conversation partner. 'Representation gestures' as their name suggests, represent a given object or action and may be considered symbolic with the meaning transferable across contexts, for example a cupped hand moved toward the mouth to represent 'drink' and may occur in the absence of the given referent. This type of gesture emerges slightly later than deictic gestures although the two frequently co-occur. Thus, at the prelinguistic stage infants are making sense of, and producing functional communication in, a number of modalities. Furthermore, studies of the relationship between gesture and spoken words indicate that children produce gestures and words as two element 'utterances' before producing two-word spoken utterances (Goldin-Meadow and Morford, 1990; Capirci, Iverson, Pizzuto and Volterra, 1996). It is suggested that this occurs as the gestural modality is more accessible when complex articulatory mechanisms are still underdeveloped compared to cognitive skills. Interestingly, the children studied did not combine two 'representation gestures' and few produced 'referential gesture and referential word' combinations which would have resulted a more complex semantic utterance, they preferred instead to do this only in the vocal mode. Capirci et al. (1996: 670) suggest this may 'reflect a deeper constraint on the gestural modality in hearing children receiving a spoken language input'. This may have implications for the potential output of children and adults who are using representational signs given the typical asymmetry of the input/output modes.

The use of keyword manual signs (with accompanying speech) would appear to capitalize upon an already naturally occurring developmental process and modality by making it more explicit and placing it within a systematic semantic framework.

Joint attention and communication development

Joint attention is known to be one of the key factors associated with successful social and communication development in all children, being based on a triadic relationship between self (infant), other (parent) and object (Bakeman and Adamson, 1984; Tomasello and Farrar, 1986; Harris, 1992; Harris, Kasari and Sigman, 1996; Moore, 1998). This becomes established, typically by 12 months, through the use of non-verbal communicative behaviours such as gesturing and pointing towards an object and checking the direction of gaze of the communication partner (Franco and Butterworth, 1996; Franco and Wishart, 1996). Typically developing infants have difficulty disengaging and shifting visual attention away from a central stimulus in the first few months and it is not until approximately 9 months of age that another's (sometimes subtle) head turn is used as cue to locate target objects (Atkinson, Hood, Wattam-Bell and Braddick 1992; Hood, 1995). The use of eye gaze as a reliable indicator for attention switch is not used typically until around 12 months and it is proposed that changes in joint visual attention might be associated with attentional control (Moore, 1998). Differences (delays) in attention switching and attention control have been observed in children with Down syndrome (Berger, 1990), as has a delay in referential looking (Ramrutten and Jenkins, 1998), and this may be one of the contributory factors to the frequently found language delay. It is possible that the more overt use of objects, sign or gesture in addition to the spoken word may highlight and facilitate joint attention for infants with Down syndrome and so help promote the language-acquisition process (Harris, Kasari and Sigman, 1996).

AAC and communication development
in Down syndrome

It is apparent from earlier (Kiernan, Reid and Jones, 1982; Layton and Savino, 1990) and more recent research findings (Grove, 1995; Launonen, 1996, 1998; see Romski and Sevcik, 1997 and Powell, 1999 for a review) that children and adults with a range of cognitive difficulties are able to develop meaningful communication through the use of AAC in the absence of intelligible speech. Miller (1992) reported that the initial vocabularies (sign and sign plus speech) of children with Down syndrome were not significantly different from their typically developing mental age-matched peers and in some cases were greater before 17 months of age, although the advantage tailed off after this time. Interestingly, the vocabularies they developed were initially different, that is, sign only, followed by sign plus speech and eventually speech only, which may indicate an early separation of the modality lexicons. This finding also supports the multimodal argument described earlier when increased proficiency in one modality leads to a reduction in the use of another that is perceived as being less efficient. This also supports the early use of sign as a temporary expedient whilst spoken language is being mastered (Launonen, 1996, 1998).

The use of AAC with individuals with Down syndrome is believed to exploit an area of relative strength – the visuo-motor channel rather than the auditory-vocal channel – when it is known that profound short-term auditory memory and processing problems are likely to exist (Bower and Hayes, 1994; Broadley, MacDonald and Buckley, 1995; Jarrold, Baddeley and Phillips, 1999). This is based upon the premiss that visual information, such as a manual sign, is more 'concrete' and accessible than the auditory trace of a spoken word, which is a transient, arbitrary sensory stimulus requiring processing and rehearsal to become a cognitive representation (Gathercole and Baddeley, 1993; Morgan Barrie, 1995). In light of this the use of graphic symbols for comprehension and expression may have an additional advantage, placing even less demand on both working memory (Iacono, Mirenda and Beukleman, 1993) and motoric generation and is believed to provide greater support for the emergence of communication than either manual signs (Iacono and Duncum, 1995) or speech (Remington and Clarke, 1996). In particular, both high- and low-technology communication aids are believed to offer positive contributions because symbols are:

- visual and concrete
- permanent and generally static
- easy to recognize and are very similar to the objects they represent – they are highly iconic and therefore can be learned quickly
- low in demands on motor skills
- supportive of early reading skills and where a voice output is attached provide verbal feedback (Murray-Branch and Gamradt, 1999).

In terms of discriminating information through a predominantly visual mode, children appear consistently able to distinguish communicative gestures from noncommunicative gestures at an early age and in multilayered linguistic organization (Pettito, 1993). This illustrates the natural multimodal nature of early communication. This differentiation for semantic qualities has also been supported for visual graphic symbols, shown in differences in recordings of auditory evoked responses (AER) in the left hemisphere frontal and temporal lobes, when children with learning difficulties were shown meaningful and nonmeaningful graphic symbols (Molfese, Morris and Romski, 1990).

Research from adults with Down syndrome suggests an additional possible explanation for the preference for visually presented stimuli: atypical cerebral organization of function for speech perception (Elliott and Weeks, 1993; Elliott, Pollock, Chua and Weeks, 1995). Adults with Down syndrome were found to be less successful than controls with learning difficulties on tasks requiring a series of movements to be performed in response to verbal instruction, however they outperformed controls when provided with a visual demonstration. This difference was attributed to the right hemisphere atypically subserving receptive speech *and* visual-spatial processing within which coexistence speech processing is disadvantaged. It may be that the comparative strength of visual over auditory information may be a result of this.

In summary, AAC has the potential to optimize communication by capitalizing on specific aspects of typically occurring multimodal development and minimizing areas of deficit by allowing meaningful communication and reinforcement of basic language concepts (Kumin, 1994) in the absence of intelligible speech.

Can AAC constrain language development?

Despite the success of manual signing (and graphic symbols) in facilitating *communication*, many AAC users with learning difficulties rarely develop *expressive language* in either mode beyond a basic level (Udwin and Yule, 1990; Grove, Dockerell and Woll, 1996; Heim and Baker-Mills, 1996; Smith, 1996a, 1996b). The reason for this has yet to be established. There are several possibilities: properties inherent in the way AAC systems are represented mentally (Hjelmquist, 1997); constraints that exist within the systems themselves (Smith, 1996a; Smith and Grove in press); the way AAC is presented as input by primarily oral communicators (Grove and McDougall, 1991); or whether different intervention strategies and modalities should be pursued at different points in the language development process (Møller and von Tetzchner, 1996). A number of these issues are explored briefly below.

Influence of the communication environment and communication partners

In the early 1970s it was recognized that whilst signs and symbols could be acquired by communicatively and cognitively impaired individuals, unless AAC was used in all contexts by communication partners it failed to enhance interaction or communicative ability (Kopchick, Rombach and Smilovitz, 1975). Despite this early acknowledgment, individuals relying upon manual signs and graphic symbols are still frequently exposed to their use only in planned routines and limited contexts, resulting in input which is both impoverished (Bryen and McGinley, 1991; Grove and McDougall, 1991; Kiernan, Reid and Jones, 1982), asymmetrical (Smith and Grove, 1996) and context specific. Studies with children (Grove and McDougall, 1991) and adults have shown decreased sign use in contexts where staff do not sign against those where they do, despite poor levels of speech intelligibility and frequent communication breakdown (Calculator and Delaney, 1986; Powell and Clibbens, 1994). In terms of input strategies, individuals developing language through AAC rarely experience the type of adjustments or 'scaffolding' in their primary (non-speech) mode that occur in typical adult–child conversations such as modelling, recasting and expansion of utterances (McTear, 1985). These strategies are believed to be key to the acquisition of higher-level morph-ology and syntax, particularly in children whose mean length of utterance (MLU) is above 2.5 (Yoder Kaiser, Goldstein et al., 1995): interestingly, the point beyond which very few AAC users progress (Grove et al, 1996; Grove and Smith in press). The point has also been made that the ability to use representational combinations beyond a one-element level in a modality may depend upon exposure to that as an input (Capirci, Iverson, Pizzuto and Volterra, 1996). The lack of opportunities to experience this may be one explanation for the paucity of more complex spontaneous utterance production (Udwin and Yule, 1991).

Socio-linguistic aspects of AAC

Who uses AAC, when, and where, can have a positive or negative impact upon AAC users, as noted above. Woll and Barnett (1998) explore this from a socio-linguistic/multilingual perspective by looking at the communities of users and the relative status of the different systems (or modalities). Communities of users are defined by the presence, or absence, of the individual's AAC modality thus: endogenous – communities where all modalities are present in all social environments; exogenous – where one/more of the modalities are not used in all social environments; and heterogeneous – where a variety of modalities are used, some of which are known, and some of which are not. The relative status of different modalities is addressed in a vertical and horizontal framework where some are seen as being hierarchically valued (additive) or devalued (subtractive) by others. An example of a subtractive situation is the use of keyword signing by adults with learning disabilities in resource centres; if staff do not sign, an asymmetry arises in modality use with clients feeling their communication mode is devalued. This is likened to the 'linguistic oppression' experienced by speakers of minority languages which leads to a reduction in the desire to interact and integrate with users of a language (Gardner and Lambert, 1972). This has a direct effect on both the use and continued learning of the language and cannot be discounted in the context of AAC acquisition and subsequent levels of competence attained. It also relates directly to the parental concerns of additional stigmatism outlined earlier (Parsons and Wills, 1992).

Strategies for teaching and learning

Behavioural changes have been noted in the acquisition of vocabulary and use of AAC (Udwin and Yule, 1990) but there is little empirical evidence suggesting the best strategies to use in intervention to support generalization (Schlosser and Lee, 2000) and spontaneous use (Carter, Hotchkis, and Cassar, 1996). To be truly effective, intervention programmes need to address acquisition, generalization and spontaneous use. The role of AAC for individuals with Down syndrome should also be considered as being responsive, multipurpose and multimodal and changing over time as different modalities are required to best serve different needs (Møller and Von Tetzchner, 1996). Initially gesture and signing may help establish dynamic social exchanges and later, in conjunction with symbols to support literacy, access to the educational curriculum, and independent living skills.

Context appears to be one of the most critical factors in AAC at both the micro level of facilitating joint attention between communication partners (utterance context) and at a macro level of use by the broader communication communities (ecological context).

Joint attention

As already discussed, joint attention is a key factor in positively influencing early vocabulary acquisition (Tomasello and Farrar, 1986; Harris, 1992). Research with children with Down syndrome has demonstrated a positive effect on receptive language when caregivers maintain joint attention, particularly when this is on a toy or object selected by the child (Harris, Kasari and Sigman, 1996). One of the reasons suggested for this is that it limits the possible range of referents available to the child in terms of matching vocabulary to the current nonverbal focus of attention. It is also believed to reduce the cognitive load and increase the likelihood of an association being made between the spoken word and the referent (Bruner, 1975; Snow, 1984). The strategies suggested to capitalize on this when using AAC (in this case keyword signs) are based on research conducted with deaf mothers using British Sign Language with their deaf children (Harris, Clibbens, Chasin and Tibbits, 1989). The aim of this is to enable children to perceive both the sign and spoken word relating to the nonverbal context of their attention, thereby maintaining and minimizing the attentional demand (Clibbens, Powell and Grove, 1997).

Sign within the child's existing visual field or signing space

This may mean displacing a sign from its usual canonical location so it relates directly to the child's focus of attention – for example, moving the sign for 'dog' away from the usual place close to the signer and placing it next to the picture or object within the child's visual field. This may involve sitting behind or next to the child when looking at books to allow a quick response to be made.

Sign on the child

In this case, the sign is again displaced from its typical position and produced on the child – for example, the sign for 'cat' would be made on the child's face rather than on that of the adult. This also provides the child with additional kinasthaetic information about where the sign is placed for when they make it spontaneously or in imitation later. It frequently prompts the child to touch the same place (anecdotal evidence) and may therefore act as a form of modelling.

Iconicity and AAC

The level of iconicity or translucency of a manual sign or graphic symbol has long been considered an important factor in the selection of initial vocabulary for individuals with learning difficulties, the belief being that the degree of representativeness would positively affect the learning process (Romski and Sevcik, 1997). However, it is now considered that this may not be the most important factor in sign or symbol acquisition, although it is acknowledged that initial vocabularies function primarily as requests for concrete referents (Schlosser, Lloyd and McNaughton, 1996).

A positive factor influencing sign or symbol acquisition is whether it is introduced to represent a word that is already within an individual's receptive vocabulary. In such instances iconicity has been shown to be of benefit (Hurlbut, Iwata and Green, 1982 cited in Schlosser, Lloyd and McNaughton, 1996). However, where receptive vocabulary is being taught through AAC this may be less relevant.

Iconicity has also been shown to have a positive effect upon listeners' perception of speech intelligibility of adults with learning difficulties using manual signs (Powell and Clibbens, 1994). Naïve listeners (with no prior knowledge of manual sign) consistently rated single words accompanied by iconic signs, but without contextual clues (edited from connected speech), as being more intelligible than those which were not accompanied by signs or when the signs were abstract in nature. This suggests that signing might assist effective communication even for listeners without sign knowledge, as many functional signs are highly iconic.

Generalization

There is now a consensus that generalization and maintenance of AAC need to be an integral part of the intervention process from the onset (Light, 1999; Schlosser and Lee, 2000) rather than an 'add on' once vocabulary has been introduced. This is particularly important for individuals with Down syndrome, where generalization and maintenance of newly acquired skills can be problematic. The implication for the style of delivery of intervention strategies, in particular those that are pragmatic and functionally relevant from the start, is that a context-based approach is required that allows frequent opportunities for rehearsal, use and reinforcement.

Communication partners and the wider communication context

The majority of earlier intervention studies focused on changing and facilitating the communicative behaviours and modalities of individuals with communication difficulties with little evidence of how communication partners were involved in the reciprocal process (Schlosser and Lee, 2000). This suggests that the shared responsibility and transactional nature of communicative exchanges have not been addressed as a matter of course in programmes of intervention, despite authors emphasizing the importance of training communication partners, particularly in the field of graphic symbol use (Cumley and Beukelman, 1992; Light, Binger, Agate and Ramsey, 1999). The importance of bimodal input (sign or symbol plus speech) by communication partners cannot be overemphasized from the perspective of modelling and promoting a shared communication mode (Calculator, 1988; Grove and McDougall, 1991; Romski and Sevcik, 1997) and in light of the socio-linguistic implications outlined earlier (Woll and Barnett, 1998).

Semantic development

There is evidence to suggest that children whose primary mode is visuospatial are able to modify signs and gestures creatively to indicate contrastive meaning even at a one-word level and, as such, may perform linguistic, non-linguistic and meta-linguistic functions (Grove, Dockrell and Woll, 1996; Grove, 1997). The importance here relies on the correct interpretation of the child's intention by the communication partner. Hence closer and more detailed analysis of *how* manual signs are produced by individuals in different contexts needs to be included in programmes of intervention rather than, as previously, noting whether signs are simply present or absent (Grove, 1990, 1997).

Conclusion

Augmentative and alternative communication should be viewed as having many purposes in its role of promoting and maintaining communication development in individuals with Down syndrome, both within and across individuals, and should not be seen as being limited in time, context or function. Longitudinally it may be used to:

- enhance prelinguistic interactions and early pragmatic skills including turn-taking and joint attention
- increase early comprehension
- enhance parent–child interactions by providing a meaningful symbolic representation of ideas beyond the immediate context
- provide a means by which children can facilitate adult speech to provide a model
- enhance the ability to be an active rather than passive conversation partner
- facilitate expressive vocabulary acquisition (with and in the absence of speech)
- support literacy development
- enhance speech intelligibility
- support the development of independent living skills.

References

Atkinson J, Hood B, Wattam-Bell J, Braddick O (1992) Changes in infants' ability to switch visual attention during the first three months of life. Perception 21: 643–53.

Bakeman R, Adamson LB (1984) Coordinating attention of people and objects in mother–infant and peer–infant interaction. Child Development 55: 1278–89.

Berger J (1990) Interactions between parents and their infants with Down syndrome. In D Cicchetti, M Beeghly (eds) Down syndrome: a developmental perspective. New York: Cambridge University Press, pp. 101–46.

Beukelman DR, Mirenda P (1998) Augmentative and Alternative Communication: Management of Severe Communication Disorders in Children and Adults. 2 edn. Baltimore: Brookes.

Bliss C (1965) Semantography (Blissymbolics). Sydney: Semantography Publications.

Bower A, Hayes A (1994) Short-term memory deficits and Down's syndrome: a comparative study. Down's Syndrome: Research and Practice 2(2): 47–50.

Broadley I, MacDonald J, Buckley S (1995) Working memory in children with Down's syndrome. Down's Syndrome: Research and Practice 3(1): 3–8.

Bruner JS (1975) The ontogenesis of speech acts. Journal of Child Language 2: 10–19.

Bryen DN, McGinley V (1991) Sign language input to community residents with SPMR: how effective is it? Education and Training of the Mentally Retarded 23: 129–37.

Buckley S (1993) Language development in children with Down syndrome: reasons for optimism. Down's Syndrome: Research and Practice 1: 3–9.

Calculator S (1988) Promoting the acquisition and generalization of conversation skills by individuals with severe disabilities. Augmentative and Alternative Communication 4: 94–103.

Calculator SN, Delaney D (1986) Comparison of nonspeaking and speaking mentally retarded adults' clarification strategies. Journal of Speech and Hearing Disorders 51: 252–9.

Capirci O, Iverson JM, Pizzuto E, Volterra V (1996) Gestures and words during the transition to two-word speech. Journal of Child Language 23: 645–73.

Carter M, Hotchkis GD, Cassar MC (1996) Spontaneity of augmentative and alternative communication in persons with intellectual disabilities: critical review. AAC Augmentative and Alternative Communication 12: 97–109.

Chapman R (1997) Language development in children and adolescents with Down syndrome. Mental Retardation and Developmental Disabilities Research Reviews 3: 307–12.

Clibbens J, Powell G, Grove N (1997) Manual signing and AAC: Issues for Research and Practice. Communication Matters 11(2): 17–18.

Cobo-Lewis A, Kimbrough Oller D, Lynch M, Levine S (1996) Relations of motor and vocal milestones in typically developing infants and infants with Down syndrome. American Journal on Mental Retardation 100(5): 456–67.

Cumley GD, Beukelman DR (1992) Roles and responsibilities of facilitators in augmentative and alternative communication. Seminars in Speech and Language 13: 111–18.

Elliott D, Weeks DJ (1993) Cerebral specialization for speech perception and movement organization in adults with Down's syndrome. Cortex 29: 103–13.

Elliott D, Pollock BJ, Chua R, Weeks DJ (1995) Cerebral specialization for spatial processing in adults with Down syndrome. American Journal on Mental Retardation 99(6): 605–15.

Foreman P, Crews G (1998) Using augmentative communication with infants and young children with Down syndrome. Down's Syndrome: Research and Practice 5(1): 16–25.

Fowler A (1990) Language abilities in children with Down's syndrome: Evidence for a specific language delay. In D Cicchetti and M Beeghly (eds) Down Syndrome: A Developmental Perspective. New York: Cambridge University Press, pp. 302–28.

Fowler A, Gelman R, Gleitman L (1994) The course of language learning in children with Down's syndrome. In H Tager-Flusberg (ed.) Constraints on Language Acquisition. Studies of Atypical Children. Hillside NJ: Erlbaum, pp. 91–140.

Franco F, Butterworth G (1996) Pointing and social awareness: declaring and requesting in the second year. Journal of Child Language 23: 307–36.

Franco F, Wishart J (1996) Preverbal communication in young children with Down's syndrome: the use of pointing and other gestures. In M Aldridge (ed.) Child Language. Clevedon: Multilingual Matters, pp. 52–64.

Gardner RC, Lambert WE (1972) Attitude and motivation in second language learning. Rowley Mass: Newbury House.

Gathercole SE, Baddeley AD (1993) Working Memory and Language. Hove: Erlbaum.

Goldin-Meadow S, Morford M (1990) Gesture in early child language. In V Volterra, CJ Erting (eds) From Gesture to Language in Hearing and Deaf Children. New York: Springer-Verlag, pp. 249–62.

Grove N (1990) Developing intelligible signs with learning disabled students: a review of the literature and an assessment procedure. British Journal of Communication Disorders 20: 265–93.

Grove N (1995) Linguistic skills of children using manual signs. Unpublished PhD dissertation, Institute of Education, University of London.

Grove N (1997) Gesture, language and multimodality: Implications for research and practice. In E Bjorck-Akesson, P Lindsay (eds) Communication . . . Naturally: Theoretical and Methodological issues in Augmentative and Alternative Communication. Proceedings of the Fourth ISAAC Research Symposium. Västerås, Sweden: Malardalen University Press, pp. 92–101.

Grove N, Dockerell J, Woll B (1996) The two-word stage in manual signs: language development in signers with intellectual impairments. In S von Tetzchner, MH Jensen (eds) Augmentative and Alternative Communication: European Perspectives. London: Whurr, pp. 101–18.

Grove N, McDougall S (1991) Exploring sign use in two settings. British Journal of Special Education 18: 149–56.

Grove N, Walker M (1990) The Makaton Vocabulary: Using signs and symbols to develop interpersonal communication. Augmentative and Alternative Communication 6: 15–28.

Harris M (1992) Language Experience and Early Language Development. Hove: Erlbaum.

Harris M, Clibbens J, Chasin J, Tibbits R (1989) The social context of early sign language development. First Language 9: 81–97.

Harris S, Kasari C, Sigman M (1996) Joint attention and language gains in children with Down syndrome. American Journal on Mental Retardation 6: 608–19.

Heim M, Baker-Mills A (1996) Early development of symbolic communication and linguistic complexity through augmentative and alternative communication. In S von Tetzchner, MH Jensen (eds) Augmentative and Alternative Communication: European Perspectives. London: Whurr, pp. 232–48.

Hjelmquist E (1997) Issues of representation in alternative language development. In R Huxley, E Ingram (eds) Language Acquisition: Models and Methods. New York: Academic Press, pp. 19–25.

Hood B (1995) Shifts of visual attention in the human infant: a neuroscientific approach. In C Rover-Collier, L Lipsett (eds) Advances in Infancy Research. Oxford: Oxford University Press, pp. 63–216.

Iacono T, Mirenda P, Beukleman D (1993) Comparison of unimodal and multi-modal AAC techniques for children with intellectual disabilities. Augmentative and Alternative Communication 9: 83–94.

Iacono T, Duncum J (1995) Comparison of sign alone and in combination with an electronic communication device in early language intervention: Case study. Augmentative and Alternative Communication 11: 249–59.

Jarrold C, Baddeley A, Phillips C (1999) Down syndrome and the phonological loop: the evidence for, and importance of, a specific verbal short-term memory deficit. Down's Syndrome: Research and Practice 6(2): 61–75.

Jenkins C (1993) Expressive language delay in children with Down's syndrome: a specific cause for concern. Down's Syndrome: Research and Practice 1(1): 10–14.

Kates B, McNaughton S (1975) The First Application of Blissymbolics as a Communication Medium for Non-speaking Children: Historical Development. Don Mills, Ontario: ESCI.

Kiernan C, Reid B, Jones L (1982) Signs and Symbols: Use of Non-vocal Communication Systems. London: Heinemann.

Kopchick GA, Rombach DW, Smilovitz R (1975) A total communication environment in an institution. Mental Retardation 13: 22–3.

Kumin L (1994) Communication skills in children with Down syndrome: a guide for parents. Rockville Md: Woodville House.

Launonen K (1996) Enhancing communication skills of children with Down syndrome: Early use of manual signs. In S von Tetzchner, MH Jensen (eds) Augmentative and Alternative Communication: European Perspectives. London: Whurr, pp. 213–30.

Launonen K (1998) Early manual sign intervention: eight year follow-up of children with Down syndrome. ISAAC Dublin 1998, 24–27 August, UCD, Dublin Ireland. Proceedings. Dublin: Ashfield Publications, pp. 371–2.

Layton TL, Savino MA (1990) Acquiring a communication system by sign and speech in a child with Down syndrome: a longitudinal investigation. Child Language Teaching and Therapy 6: 59–76.

LeProvost P (1983) Using the Makaton Vocabulary in early language training with a Down's baby: a single case study. Mental Handicap 11: 28–9.

LeProvost P (1993) The use of signing to encourage first words. In S Buckley, M Emslie, G Haslegrave, P LeProvost (eds) The Development of Language and Reading Skills in Children with Down's Syndrome. Portsmouth: University of Portsmouth.

Light J (1999) Do augmentative and alternative communication interventions really make a difference? The challenges of efficacy research. Augmentative and Alternative Communication 15: 13–24.

Light J, Binger C, Agate TL, Ramsey KN (1999) Teaching partner-focused questions to individuals who use augmentative and alternative communication to enhance their communicative competence. Journal of Speech, Language, and Hearing Research 42: 241–55.

Lynch MP, Kimbrough Oller D, Steffens ML, Levine SL, Basinger DL, Umbel V (1995) Onset of speech-like vocalisations in infants with Down syndrome. American Journal on Mental retardation 100(1): 68–86.

McTear M (1985) Children's Conversation. Oxford: Basil Blackwell.

Miller J (1992) Development of speech and language in children with Down syndrome. In IT Lott, EE McCoy (eds) Down Syndrome: Advances in Medical Care. Chichester: Wiley-Liss.

Molfese D, Morris RD, Romski, MA (1990) Semantic discrimination in nonspeaking youngsters with moderate or severe retardation: electro-physiological correlates. Brain and Language 38: 61–74.

Møller S, Von Tetzchner S (1996) Allowing for developmental potential: a case study of intervention change. In S von Tetzchner, MH Jensen (eds) Augmentative and Alternative Communication: European Perspectives. London: Whurr, pp. 249–69.

Moore C (1998) Gaze-following and the control of attention. In P Rochat (ed.), Early Social Cognition. Hillside New Jersey: Erlbaum.

Morgan Barrie R (1995) Observing and assessing auditory skills in children. In S Wirtz (ed.) Perceptual Approaches to Communication Disorders. London: Whurr.

Murray-Branch JE, Gamradt JE (1999) Assistive technology: strategies and tools for enhancing the communication skills of children with Down syndrome. In J Millar, M Leddy, L Leavitt (eds) Improving the Communication of People with Down Syndrome. London: Brookes, Chapter 9.

Parsons C, Wills J (1992) Parental compliance with recommendations to utilise augmentative communication with their children with Down syndrome. Australian Journal of Human Communication Disorders 2: 1–19.

Pettito L (1993) Modularity and constraints in early lexical acquisition: evidence from children's early language and gesture. In P Bloom (ed.) Language acquisition: core readings. London: Harvester Wheatsheaf, pp. 95–126.

Powell G (1999) Current research findings to support the use of signs with adults and children with intellectual and communication difficulties. Presented at MVDP International Tutors Conference, University of Surrey, August.

Powell G, Clibbens J (1994) Actions speak louder than words: signing and speech intelligibility in adults with Down's syndrome. Down's Syndrome: Research and Practice 2: 127–9.

Ramrutten B, Jenkins C (1998) Prelinguistic communication and Down syndrome. Down's Syndrome: Research and Practice 5(2): 53–62.

Remington B, Clarke S (1996) Alternative and augmentative systems of communication for children with Down's syndrome. In J Rondal, J Perera, L Nadel, A Comblain (eds) Down's Syndrome: Psychological, Psychobiological and Socioeducational Perspectives. London: Whurr, pp. 129–43.

Romski MA, Sevcik RA (1997) Augmentative and alternative communication for children with developmental disabilities. Mental Retardation and Developmental Disabilities Research Reviews 3: 363–8.

Rondal J (1995) Exceptional language development in Down syndrome. Implications for the cognition–language relationship. New York: Cambridge University Press.

Rondal J (1996) Oral language in Down's syndrome. In J Rondal, J Perera, L Nadel, A Comblain (eds) (1996) Down' Syndrome: Psychological, psychobiological and socio-educational perspectives. London: Whurr, pp. 99–117.

Rondal J, Perera J, Nadel L, Comblain A (eds) (1996) Down's Syndrome: Psychological, Psychobiological and Socio-educational Perspectives. London: Whurr.

Roy DM, Panayi M (1997) Gesture and motor impairment. In E Bjorck-Akesson, P Lindsay (eds) Communication . . . Naturally: Theoretical and Methodological Issues in Augmentative and Alternative Communication. Proceedings of the Fourth ISAAC Research Symposium. Västerås, Sweden: Malardalen University Press, pp. 67–75.

Schlosser RW, Lloyd LL, McNaughton S (1996) Graphic symbol selection in research and practice: making the case for a goal-driven process. In E Bjork-Akesson and P Lindsay (eds) Communication . . . Naturally: Theoretical and Methodological Issues in Augmentative and Alternative Communication. Proceedings of the Fourth ISAAC Research Symposium. Västerås, Sweden: Malardalen University Press, pp. 126–39.

Schlosser RW, Lee DL (2000) Promoting generalization and maintenance in augmentative and alternative communication: a meta-analysis of 20 years of effectiveness research. AAC Augmentative and Alternative Communication 16: 208–26.

Schmidt-Sidor B, Wisniewski KE, Shepard TH, Sersen EA (1990) Brain growth in Down syndrome subjects 15 to 22 weeks of gestational age, and birth to 60 months. Clinical Neuropathology 9: 181–90.

Schweigert PD, Rowland C (1998) Tangible Symbols: Concrete Bridge to Abstract Communication in Autism and Severe Disabilities. Paper presented at ISAAC Dublin 1998, 24–27 August, UCD, Dublin, Ireland.

Sisson LA, Barrett RP (1984) An alternative treatments comparison of oral and total communication training with minimally verbal retarded children. Journal of Applied Behaviour Analysis 17: 559–66.

Smith M (1996a) The medium or the message: a study of speaking children using communication boards. In S von Tetzchner, MH Jensen (eds) Augmentative and Alternative Communication: European Perspectives. London: Whurr, pp. 119–36.

Smith M (1996b) The bimodal situation of children developing alternative modes of language. Paper presented to the Fourth Research Symposium of the International Society of Augmentative and Alternative Communication, Vancouver, Canada, August.

Smith M (1997) The bimodal situation of children developing alternative modes of language. In E Bjorck-Akesson, P Lindsay (eds), Communication . . . Naturally: Theoretical and Methodological Issues in Augmentative and Alternative Communication. Proceedings of the Fourth ISAAC Research Symposium. Västerås, Sweden: Malardalen University Press, pp. 12–18.

Smith M, Grove N (1996) Input/output asymmetries: Implications for language development in AAC. Paper presented at 7th Biennial Conference of the International Society for Augmentative and Alternative Communication, Vancouver, Canada. August 7–10th.

Snow C (1984) Parent–child interaction and the development of communicative ability. In RL Schiefelbusch, J Pickar (eds) The Acquisition of Communicative Competence. Baltimore: University Park Press, pp. 69–107.

Stoel-Gammon C (1997) Phonological development in Down syndrome. Mental Retardation and Developmental Disabilities Research Reviews 3: 300–6.

Tomasello M, Farrar MJ (1986) Joint attention and early language. Child Development 57: 1454–63.

Udwin O, Yule W (1990) Augmentative communication systems taught to cerebral palsy children – a longitudinal study. 1. The acquisition of signs and symbols, and syntactic aspects over time. British Journal of Disorders of Communication 25: 295–309.

Udwin O, Yule W (1991) Augmentative communication systems taught to cerebral palsy children – a longitudinal study. 3: teaching practices and exposure to sign and symbol use in schools and homes. British Journal of Disorders of Communication 26: 149–62.

Von Tetzchner S, Jensen MH (eds.) (1996) Augmentative and Alternative Communication: European Perspectives. London: Whurr.

Walker M (1976) The Makaton Vocabulary (Revised). London: Royal Association in Aid of the Deaf and Dumb.

Walker M, Parson P, Cousins S, Carpenter B, Park K (1985) Symbols for Makaton. Back Hill, UK: Earo, The Resource Centre.

Woll B, Barnett S (1998) Towards a sociolinguistic perspective on augmentative and alternative communication. AAC Augmentative and Alternative Communication 14: 200–11.

Yoder PJ, Kaiser AP, Goldstein H, Alpert C, Mousetis L, Kaczmarek L, Fischer R (1995). An exploratory comparison of milieu teaching and responsive interaction in classroom applications. Journal of Early Intervention 19: 218–42.

Zangari C, Lloyd L, Vicker B (1994) Augmentative and alternative communication: an historic perspective. Augmentative and Alternative Communication 10: 27–59.

Chapter 9
Literacy and language

SUE BUCKLEY

Introduction

The aim of this chapter is to draw attention to the importance of reading instruction and involvement in literacy for developing the spoken language skills of children, teenagers and adults with Down syndrome. The opportunity to learn to read and to be involved in reading activities is important for two main reasons, in order to acquire a useful level of literacy skills and in order to improve spoken language. Many more children with Down syndrome are acquiring literacy skills than was the case 15 years ago and early exposure to reading activities may be one of the most effective ways to improve the grammar and phonology of their spoken language.

This chapter reviews the evidence for:

- the range of literacy skills being gained by children and teenagers with Down syndrome at the present time
- the benefits of literacy instruction for speech, language and memory skills
- effective teaching methods which link literacy and speech and language goals
- the role of the speech and language therapist in supporting literacy teaching.

The range of literacy skills

It is probably still appropriate to say that there is very little information available to provide an accurate guide to the range of literacy achievements that can be expected for a representative population of children and teenagers with Down syndrome, as many children still do not receive effective literacy instruction in their schools. However, data from a number of studies are beginning to provide some useful information.

Studies from Australia and New Zealand report on small samples of children followed up from early intervention programmes. For a group of eight children with Down syndrome followed up from the Macquarie Programme, Sydney (chronological age 7;2 to 9;3 and IQ 48 to 67), reading ages of 6;1 to 9;3 are reported (Pieterse and Center, 1984; Pieterse, 1988). Some of the children from this early intervention group are included in a study of the literacy skills of 30 Australian adults (Bochner, Outhred and Pieterse, 2001). This study reports on the reading and language achievements of individuals from age 18 to 36 years, with most of them being between 18 and 24 years. The average reading ability of the group, measured with a reading assessment which taps all aspects of reading skills, was 8;1, range 6;7 to 11;0. Those over 24 years had lower achievements than the younger individuals, who had experienced better educational opportunities. Only one individual could not score at all on the task. The average reading score was higher for those who had been in mainstream education, 8;9 compared with 7;7 for those from special education settings. However, of the 14 'very good, fluent and expressive' readers (p. 82), seven were from mainstream and seven from special education. These fluent text readers are also reported to have good, intelligible spoken language suggesting a benefit of reading activity for speech and language, but longitudinal studies are needed to establish the nature of the relationship. Overall, speech clarity and intelligibility was better for the adults who had been in inclusive education settings, supporting the similar findings of Buckley, Bird, Sacks and Archer (2002, in press). Those in inclusive settings have the benefit of communicating with peers with typical speech and language, as well as more intensive reading instruction.

Only four of the 30 Australian adults could not attempt the text reading task. The average language comprehension score for the group on a vocabulary test was 7;2, with two very high scorers achieving scores of 17;8 and 16;6. The authors note that the whole group showed interest in reading and drawing activities during leisure time. Two of the group had been actors in a TV series and had learned their scripts, with reading and language ages between 8 and 10 years. The best readers had the best language scores and the individuals who had been introduced to reading in preschool had the highest reading scores as adults. This added benefit of early reading is also confirmed in the author's work and discussed further later in this chapter.

Irwin (1989) reports on the progress of 21 children with Down syndrome, chronological age (CA) 9;6 to 11;6, in New Zealand. Nine could score on a standardized reading test (Neale Analysis of Reading Ability) with scores ranging from 7;3 to 10;0 on reading accuracy. Their Stanford Binet IQs ranged from 36 to 63, their mean vocabulary comprehension age on the Peabody Picture Vocabulary Test was 4;5 with scores ranging from 2;9 to 6;7. In these studies the reader will note that reading appears to be a particular strength and that reading abilities are better than would be predicted from IQ or language measures.

Fowler, Doherty and Boynton (1995) report data on the language and literacy skills of a group of young adults in the USA who were recruited because they had good literacy skills in order to explore the links between these skills and their language and short-term memory skills. For 33 young adults with Down syndrome, aged 17 to 25 years, Fowler reports reading ages of 5;7 to 16;0 for word attack skills, 6;7 to 12;7 for word identification and 5;6 to 8;4 for reading comprehension. These young people had mental ages of 5;0 to 7;1, vocabulary ages of 6;1 to 11;1 and grammar ages of 5;1 to 7;8. The reader will note that reading comprehension is close to grammar comprehension and word identification close to vocabulary age. Reading performances all range above that which might be predicted from mental age measures.

In a survey of 90 teenagers in the UK (Buckley and Sacks, 1987) parents reported that 66 of the teenagers could read at least a 'social sight' vocabulary. Of these 66 readers, just half could read more than 50 words and 15 (16% of the total group) could be described as quite good readers and enjoyed reading books, including adventure stories and books on sport or nature. In this study, many parents commented that their teenagers attempted to master the TV, sport and pop music pages of the newspaper and that even those unable to read, enjoyed being read to and looking at books. Carr and Hewitt (1982), reporting on a group of 43 individuals aged 16 years in the UK, states that seven could read quite well, about the same proportion of the group as in the 1987 study.

The author and colleagues (Buckley, 1985; Buckley and Bird, 1993; Buckley, Bird and Byrne, 1996a) have reported a number of case studies indicating a wide range of progress and often exceptional progress for children who begin learning to read at 2 to 3 years of age. For example, Joni at CA 10;4 has a reading age of 10;10 (British Ability Scales, BASI), spelling age 9;5 (BASI) and reading comprehension of 7;3 (Wechsler Objective Reading Dimensions, WORD). She can write short stories with no assistance, including stories containing the speech of characters. She writes fully grammatically correct English. Her vocabulary comprehension is 6;3 (BPVS), her grammar comprehension is 6;8 (Test for Reception of Grammar, TROG) and she uses a range of complete sentence structures in her expressive language, including correct verb tense markers, conjunctions and auxiliary verbs. Her articulation and phonology are also exceptionally good for a child with Down syndrome and she has a digit span of 4. (For examples of her written work see Buckley, 2001.) The author knows of a number of other early readers who, like Joni, have exceptional spoken and written language skills at 10 or 11 years. Recent case studies provided by parents (Dickinson, 2002; Kotlinski and

Kotlinski, 2002; Rozen, 2002; Oke, 2002) describe similar features in their children's early reading progress. Their children were all introduced to reading instruction when at the beginning stage of vocabulary acquisition and they all describe faster than typical learning. In particular, they note that reading was not only an easy and enjoyable activity, it promoted both expressive grammar and phonology – their children used complete sentences much earlier than is expected for children with Down syndrome and they spoke more clearly. The link between improved phonology and grammar could be explained by Locke's view that as a child begins to try to express inflectional morphology (for example 'ing', 'ed', 's' endings) this promotes more sophisticated control in phonology (Locke, 1994, 1997). The child not attempting to express grammar may be missing a phase that is important for the development of phonology.

One of these early reading children, Charlotte, was assessed by the first author at the age of 5;0. She was introduced to reading at 2;6 when she had some 30–40 spoken words. She had not begun to combine words at this point. At 5;0 years of age, Charlotte's vocabulary comprehension (BPVS) was 4;10 and her grammar comprehension (TROG) 5;6. In her expressive language Charlotte was using complete sentences, with articles, prepositions, pronouns, auxiliaries, and correct verb tense markers. Charlotte's progress is particularly good, but in the author's experience, she is representative of the group of children whose parents effectively implement early reading to teach spoken language.

Some studies of larger and more representative samples of children with Down syndrome in mainstream education have begun to take place in the UK (Appleton, Buckley and MacDonald, 2002; Buckley, Bird and Byrne, 1996a and b; Byrne, 1997; Byrne, Buckley, MacDonald and Bird 1995; Byrne, MacDonald and Buckley, 2002).

A study of early reading compared the progress of 18 children with Down syndrome with that of age-matched typically developing peers, CA 2;0 to 4;11 mean 4;1, at the start of the study (Appleton, 2000; Appleton, Buckley and MacDonald, in press). The children were taught a sight word vocabulary by their parents under the supervision of the researchers. The progress of the two groups over the first year was very similar. After six months the average sight vocabulary learned was 15 words for the typically developing group and 17 words for the children with Down syndrome. There were large individual differences in the number of words learned in both groups, with some children learning no words and some learning 66 or 67 words, in both groups. By the third year of the study, when the average age of the children was 6;7 and they were in school, the progress of the readers in the two groups (readers are defined as those who can score on standardized reading tests) was compared. These readers (16 of 17 typically developing children and 11 of 18 children with Down syndrome) are at a similar level for reading and reading comprehension. Their scores are not significantly different and the children with Down syndrome are reading at their age level (reading BASI mean 6;7, reading comprehension Kaufman Assessment Battery mean 6;7). These data support the view that early reading skills are a significant strength for children with Down syndrome. Sixty-one per cent are keeping up with their peers at this stage in reading, despite delayed speech and language. The data provide some support for the influence of early reading for spoken language development as the readers and non-readers are not significantly different on language measures at the start of the study, but the readers make more progress over the three years, at which point they are eight months ahead on expressive language and 11 months ahead on comprehension (Reynell Developmental Language Scales). It was not possible to identify any child characteristics that distinguished the readers from the non-readers at the start of the study and variation in progress could be associated with variations in the frequency and enthusiasm of parents' teaching, but no consistent data were collected on this.

In another longitudinal study, the progress of 24 school-age children with Down syndrome – 10 girls and 14 boys, CA 4;11 to 12;7 (mean 8;2) – was evaluated and compared with the progress of a group of their non-disabled mainstream classmates who were matched with them on reading age (and were therefore slow readers for their age), as well as a group of classmates who were average readers for their age (Byrne, Buckley, MacDonald and Bird, 1995; Byrne, 1997; Byrne, MacDonald and Buckley, 2002). The study charted the reading, writing and spelling progress of the children, looking at the cognitive strategies they were using to read and the links between reading, language and memory skills. These children were fully included in the mainstream classroom and received similar literacy teaching to their peers, with the individual support of a Learning Support Assistant.

At the start of the study, all the children with Down syndrome were learning to read and their reading ages ranged from 5;0 to 8;5 for word reading (BASI), 6;0 to 7;0 for comprehension (WORD) and 6;0 to 7;2 for spelling (BASI). Vocabulary ages (BPVS) ranged from 3;7 to 5;4 and grammar ages (TROG) from 4;0 to 5;0. The children with Down syndrome had reading ages higher than their language comprehension ages would predict.

The typically developing children identified by their teachers as average readers for their age demonstrated even and age-appropriate cognitive profiles over all the measures, whereas the slower readers for their age in the same classes (matched for word reading ability to the children with Down syndrome) turned out to be significantly delayed relative to the average readers on all the language and cognitive measures (see Byrne, MacDonald, Buckley and Bird, 1995). The children with Down syndrome, while matched with the slower readers on the reading measures, were significantly behind them on number, language and memory measures. In other words, the children with Down syndrome showed advanced reading ability compared with all their other cognitive skills at this time.

By phase three of this study, two years after the first assessments, the children with Down syndrome were still not significantly behind the slow readers on word reading but they were on spelling and reading comprehension. Byrne (1997) also assessed the children's understanding and use of phonics, using their ability to read non-words as a measure of phonic (alphabetic) skills. The children were asked to read words presented on the computer screen. The children with Down syndrome were as able as the slow readers to read content and function words but, as a group, they were significantly behind the slow readers in their ability to use phonics to read non-words, so appeared to be keeping up their good word recognition skills by relying on visual memory and logographic reading (see Buckley, 2001).

However, at this point, seven of the children with Down syndrome do have alphabetical skills – they can read some nonwords correctly, demonstrating the ability to use their phonic knowledge for decoding. These children have a mean word reading age (BASI) of 7;10 range 7;4 to 9;10 (CA's 8;10 to 11;4), mean reading comprehension age (WORD) of 6;8, range 6;6 to 7;6, mean spelling age (BASI) of 7;4, range 6;9 to 8;4, mean vocabulary comprehension age (BPVS) 5;9, range 4;5 to 8;11, mean grammar comprehension age (TROG) of 5;0, range 4;6 to 5;9, mean number age (BASI) of 5;5, range 5;3 to 5;11. A further nine of the children with Down syndrome are described as logographic (sight) readers and they have mean reading, reading comprehension and spelling scores between 6 and 7 years on standardized tests. The remaining eight children with Down syndrome have reading, comprehension and spelling ages between 5 and 6 years. At this time, it is not possible to determine why some children with Down syndrome are making better progress with literacy. There was a tendency for the alphabetic children to be the older group, but the age differences between the three groups were not statistically significant (Byrne, 1997).

Four years from the start of this study, 17 children with Down syndrome, still in mainstream schools and in the research area, were followed up. At this time their chronological ages ranged from 9;2 to 14;5 (mean 11;5). Their word reading ages (BASI) range from 5;5 to 9;0 (mean 7;2), spelling ages (BASI) range from 6;1 to 9;11 (mean 7;4) reading comprehension ages (WORD) ranged from 6;0 to 7;6 (mean 6;6) vocabulary ages (BPVS) range from 3;2 to 12;2 (mean 6;0) and grammar ages (TROG) ranged from 4;0 to 5;9 (mean 5;0). Nine of these children had reading ages over 7;4, and eight of the nine had spelling ages over 7 years, with reading comprehension for the nine ranging from 6;0 to 7;6. All of the 17 children could score on standardized word reading tests, 16 could score on spelling and 14 on reading comprehension. If these data are compared to the studies carried out in the UK with earlier cohorts of children already described, then this Hampshire group was clearly achieving much higher rates of literacy acquisition than the cohorts of the 1980s or before.

These children have many more years of education in school and further education ahead of them. Half of them are showing independent reading skills at a level to give them functional literacy as adults and it is likely that 60% to 70% will reach this level by adult life.

Two conclusions may be drawn from the available evidence at this time. Some children with Down syndrome will achieve functional levels of literacy (8 years and above), others will achieve a level of literacy skill that will allow them to record work in the classroom and to read with assistance. Some may not achieve any useful level of independent literacy skills but their speech and language may benefit from literacy activities. At present the research groups are small and access to good literacy teaching is still not available to all children in the UK. Accurate estimates of what might be expected still need to be documented by studying larger samples of children.

These studies give some indication of the achievements of children with Down syndrome but it is not clear that they are representative of the whole range of ability found in a population with Down syndrome. They are reporting on children who have participated in early intervention programmes and have probably experienced better-than-average educational opportunities. It is likely that these groups do not include the children with more significant levels of developmental disability and these groups also may not be representative of all families, as the pioneering early intervention and mainstreaming programmes were often linked to universities and parents would choose to join them. Teachers, speech and language therapists and parents need to have information about the whole range of ability, as some children will learn more slowly than others and reach different levels of achievement. The author and colleagues (Buckley, Bird, Sacks and Archer, 2002, in press) recently completed a survey of a representative group of 46 teenagers, in both mainstream and special schools, in the county of Hampshire in the UK, and these data clearly show this wide range of achievement. However, before discussing the data in more detail, it should be stressed that involvement in literacy activities and in literacy instruction may benefit all children with Down syndrome, even those with the most significant cognitive and developmental difficulties as they can support language learning at all stages from first word comprehension onwards. Others have also stressed the benefits of valuing all literacy achievements (Kliewer, 1998) and of being involved in the world of literacy and storytelling (Grove, 1998).

The Hampshire group includes 18 teenagers who have received all their education in mainstream inclusive settings and 28 who have been educated in special schools, and it appears to be representative of the whole range of abilities associated with Down syndrome. Placement in the two school systems was based on where the teenagers lived, not on ability, as one part of the county began including children with Down syndrome into its local community schools before the rest of the county. The teenagers in the mainstream schools have had good daily literacy instruction from the age of 5 years or earlier, so their progress may indicate the range of achievement possible when children with Down syndrome receive the level of instruction available to other typically developing children in school. These teenagers have been fully included in the class literacy activities with a peer group the same age or one year younger, and with the individual support of a learning support assistant.

The figures in Table 9.1 illustrate the reading achievements of 41 of the teenagers and the figures in Table 9.2 illustrate their writing achievements. The figures are based on survey data from the Vineland Adaptive Behaviour Scales (VABS) and the Buckley and Sacks (1987) questionnaire used in this study.

The five 'least able' teenagers from the special schools have not been included in this comparison of outcomes from the two school systems. Children with this level of developmental disability would not have been placed in a mainstream classroom at the time these teenagers entered the school system. No one in this group had any literacy skills as a teenager but we do not know what kind of literacy experiences or instruction they have received. Two were diagnosed as autistic, none had more than 100 words or signs and three had very significant levels of behaviour difficulties. They represent 11% of this Hampshire study sample and they are a group whose needs should not be forgotten. In the earlier study in the same county (Buckley and Sacks, 1987) the percentage of teenagers with this level of difficulty was the same – 10 in a group of 90 teenagers in 1987 and five in a group of 46 teenagers in 1999.

Returning to the figures in Tables 9.1 and 9.2, it can be seen that some 80% of the teenagers in the mainstream classrooms have achieved a functional level of literacy skills and some are still in their early teenage years and can be expected to make further progress. The VABS data provide evidence of progress with age in teenage years, for receptive, expressive and written language, as illustrated in Table 9.3 (with the caution that these are cross-sectional not longitudinal data). The figures in Table 9.3 illustrate that there were no significant differences in receptive language abilities as measured by the VABS between teenagers in special or mainstream classrooms. However, there were significant differences in expressive and written language in favour of the fully included mainstream children. The author and colleagues have argued elsewhere (Buckley, Bird, Sacks and Archer, 2002; Buckley and Sacks, 2002) that there may be a link between the advanced literacy and expressive language skills of the mainstreamed children in this study. Some readers may also be interested to note that the mainstreamed children in this study have communication skills in line with their daily living and socialization skills on the VABS (see further Buckley and Sacks, 2002). Previous

American research using the same measure predicts that communication will be significantly behind the other areas for children with Down syndrome (Dyken, Hodapp and Evans, 1994). Reading is a language activity, and all reading activities have the potential to teach new vocabulary and grammar to children. Reading aloud, with or without support, provides practice for talking in complete sentences. In addition, phonics activities and spelling work may improve discrimination for speech sounds as well as for articulation and phonology. This argument is explored further in the next section.

Table 9.1. The reading skills of teenagers with Down syndrome, 11–20 years. Percentage achieving each skill (reproduced from Bird and Buckley 2002, with permission).

Reading achievements of a representative sample of teenagers with Down syndrome – 1999	Mainstream group N=18 (%)	Special school group N=23 (%)
Reading at all	100	100
Reads own name	100	83
Reads words – none	-	22
6–10	-	13
11–20	6	26
21–50	-	9
Over 50	94	30
Reads at least three common signs	94	68
Reads some social sight words	100	83
Can read sentences	100	57
Can read simple stories aloud	94	32
Can read simple stories aloud with ease	88	27
Can read books	100	39
Can read books of at least Year 2 level	94	23
Can read books of at least Year 4 level	65	9
Reads on own initiative	82	27
Reads books of at least Year 4 level on own initiative	53	9
Reads the newspaper	83	22
Can read adult newspaper stories	18	5
Reads adult newspaper stories each week	18	5
Can read instructions	94	48
Can read for pleasure	78	35
Identifies two letters found in own name	94	82
Recites all letters of the alphabet	82	27
Identifies 10 printed letters	94	50
Can name all the letters of alphabet	94	36
Knows sounds of all the letters of the alphabet	89	39
Can sound out new words when reading	78	30
Can sound out new words when spelling	72	22
Can arrange words alphabetically	59	23
Can use a dictionary	29	5
Can use a table of contents when reading	35	9
Can use an index when reading	12	9

Table 9.2. The writing skills of teenagers with Down syndrome, 11–20 years. Percentage achieving each skill (reproduced from Bird and Buckley, 2002, with permission).

Reading achievements of a representative sample of teenagers with Down syndrome – 1999	Mainstream group N=18 (%)	Special school group N=23 (%)
Can trace letters/words	94	91
Copies at least five letters from a model	88	64
Writes in cursive some of the time	59	14
Writes in cursive most of the time	53	14
Writes own first and last name	88	50
Can write own address	61	30
Can write family names	94	48
Prints or writes 10 words from memory	83	30
Prints or writes simple sentences of three or four words	82	27
Can write at least 20 words from memory	71	18
Can write more than 20 words from memory	65	18
Can write short notes or messages	71	23
Can write a simple story	61	4
Can write a short letter	61	22
Writes reports or compositions	18	-
Addresses envelopes completely	12	14
Writes advanced letters	6	-
Writes business letters	6	-

Table 9.3. Progress with age for the communication skills of teenagers with Down syndrome. Reproduced with permission from Buckley and Bird (2002).

VABS mean receptive language age Age group in years	Mainstream (N=17)	Special school (N=22)
1. 11y to 13y 11m	5y 8m	5y 0m
2. 14y to 17y 11m	5y 11m	5y 1m
3. 18 to 20y	6y 9m	6y 4m
Total group	5y 11m	5y 6m
VABS mean expressive language age Age group in years		
1. 11y to 13y 11m	4y 3m	2y 10m
2. 14y to 17y 11m	4y 11m	2y 10m
3. 18 to 20y	11y 7m	4y 1m
Total group	5y 9m	3y 3m
VABS mean written language age Age group in years		
1. 11y to 13y 11m	7y 9m	6y 7m
2. 14y to 17y 11m	8y 6m	4y 8m
3. 18 to 20y	14y 3m	6y 7m
Total group	9y 1m	5y 9m

The benefits of literacy instruction for speech, language and memory skills

The possible benefits of reading instruction for the speech and language development of children with Down syndrome was brought to the attention of the author in 1979 by Leslie Duffen, whose daughter, Sarah, had Down syndrome. Leslie wrote to the author describing how he had introduced reading to Sarah at the age of 3 years, specifically teaching her to read words and sentences that were developmentally appropriate and that she could use to talk. When he started, Sarah had very few spoken words and Leslie observed that the words that they were reading appeared in her spoken language much more quickly than words she only heard. He felt that her advanced progress (like Joni, described earlier, Sarah was speaking well, reading at almost an age-appropriate level and being educated in a mainstream school at the age of 11 years) had been due to finding that reading was the key to learning for Sarah (Duffen, 1976). Sarah could learn language more effectively from seeing it than from hearing it, suggesting that the language learning of children with Down syndrome was being held back by difficulties of accessing language in the auditory mode. More than 20 years later, the research evidence confirms that this is the case. It is now agreed that children with Down syndrome have specific speech and language impairment – that is speech and language skills significantly delayed relative to their non-verbal mental ability (Chapman, 1999; Chapman and Hesketh, 2001; Miller, 1999) One research team has data illustrating that children with specific language impairment in the general population and children with Down syndrome matched for non-verbal mental age have very similar profiles of speech, language and verbal short-term memory deficits (Laws and Bishop, 2002). Why should this be the case? It indicates that it is not simply cognitive delay that is holding back speech and language development. The evidence suggests that hearing, auditory processing and verbal short-term memory difficulties are major factors. Children with Down syndrome are at high risk for mild to moderate hearing loss, with some 80% of preschoolers suffering from conductive losses, and some of these will also have sensorineural losses (see Shott, 2000). In teenage and early adult years some 50% of the population of individuals with Down syndrome still have mild to moderate losses (see Marcell, 1995). In addition to hearing loss, there has been growing evidence for auditory short-term memory difficulties, which will compromise language processing in the auditory mode (see Conners' chapter, this volume). Recent reviews of working memory research on Down syndrome highlight the evidence for a degree of phonological loop impairment (see Jarrold, Baddeley and Phillips, 1999; Jarrold and Baddeley, 2001). Visual short-term memory spans tend to be as expected for non-verbal mental age for individuals with Down syndrome but verbal short-term memory spans are specifically impaired. A basic phonological loop impairment will affect language learning from the earliest stages, as the phonological loop is thought to hold the phonological representation (the sound pattern) of a word. This is necessary in order for the sound pattern to reach a long-term memory store and to be linked accurately to a meaning for the word. An accurate sound pattern needs to be stored in order to support the production of the spoken word in future, as well as its comprehension. Any impairment in phonological loop function will significantly affect learning to understand and say single words from infancy to adult life (Dodd and Thompson, 2001).

Research has also identified that the growth in the processing capacity of the working memory system, as measured by word or digit spans, is significantly impaired relative to the non-verbal abilities of children with Down syndrome, and this will make processing sentences and learning grammar more difficult. A number of recent studies have produced evidence to link expressive language skills and verbal short-term memory skills in children and teenagers with Down syndrome (see Chapman and Hesketh, 2001 for a review). Therefore, there is evidence to support the view that learning a language from listening will be difficult for children with Down syndrome. The hypothesis that reading may be a particularly important 'way in' to spoken language for children with Down syndrome, because it makes language visual, is therefore, plausible. However, is there any evidence that reading actually does improve their spoken language?

The author and colleagues have reported case studies of early readers since 1983 and these are indicative of the positive effects but not, perhaps, evidence to convince the sceptics. Children introduced to reading activities designed to teach spoken language, as early as 2 to 3 years of age, show significantly advanced speech, language, literacy and verbal short-term memory skills in childhood and teenage years. These children show more advanced speech, language and literacy skills as teenagers than children introduced to reading after 5 or 6 years of age. Children introduced to reading at any age after 5 years almost certainly benefit very significantly from reading activities, as has been stressed in studies reported already. However, as is demonstrated in the deaf literature (Mayberry, Lock and Kazmi, 2002), language progress in sign or speech before 5 years is very important and those starting later progress significantly but they do not catch up with the early starters. This author has argued elsewhere (Buckley, 2000), drawing on the work of Locke (1994, 1997) and others, that the brain is optimally ready to learn a first language from 12 months to 5 or 6 years. When print is used to support first language learning from 2 to 3 years of age it seems to have a qualitatively different and much greater effect, possibly as a result of brain plasticity at this age.

An experimental training study with teenagers with Down syndrome (Buckley, 1993, 1995) demonstrated that language teaching activities could significantly improve both their comprehension and production of grammar. The teaching method which used print was more effective than spoken language practice only, and the 'least able' teenagers in this special school group, non-readers at the start, showed the greatest benefit of using print. They were also found to be the students with the poorest verbal short-term memories. The methods used are described in full in Buckley (2000).

However, the first small piece of evidence of benefits of ordinary literacy instruction in school based on group data came from a longitudinal study of short-term memory development carried out by the author's research team (Laws, Buckley, Bird, MacDonald and Broadley, 1995) and discussed in detail elsewhere (Buckley, Bird and Byrne, 1996b; Buckley and Bird, 2001a, b). In this study, a group of children with Down syndrome who were learning to read over a four-year period were compared with children who were not learning to read. At the end of the period the readers were significantly ahead of the non-readers in language comprehension and verbal short-term memory measures. The gains were approximately equivalent to two years of typical developmental progress – that is, the readers were two years ahead of the non-readers on the measures, even though the two groups scored at the same level on all the measures four years earlier. This effect of reading progress for language and memory development has been demonstrated for typically developing children (Ellis and Large, 1988; Gathercole and Baddeley, 1993 a,b) and for speech and language impaired children (Stothard, Snowling, Bishop, Chipchase and Kaplan, 1998).

Some of the recent studies of reading effects for children with Down syndrome are, however, confounded by school placement effects. In the above study (Laws, Buckley, Bird, MacDonald and Broadley, 1995) all but one of the readers were in mainstream schools and all the nonreaders were in special schools in the UK. The children in the mainstream schools are in a much richer spoken language environment than the children in the special schools, where most of their peers have significant speech, language and cognitive delays. Therefore the speech and language gains may be in part due to the language environment and in part due to literacy experience and progress. In a further study of mainstream and special school outcomes, Laws, Byrne and Buckley (2000) report significantly advanced language comprehension and short-term memory skills for the mainstreamed children. Significant differences in favour of the mainstream children were reported for vocabulary comprehension, grammar comprehension, sentence memory and both auditory and visual digit span. However, although 22 of the 24 children in mainstream schools could score on a standardized reading test, only three of the 24 children in the special schools could achieve a score. Therefore the advantage for the mainstream children may be linked to reading progress but this could not be systematically explored for this study. In a follow-up study of 30 children attending special schools for children with severe learning difficulties in the UK, Laws and Gunn (2001) report an increase in reading ability over a five-year period. The number of readers (those who could read at least one word on a standard test) had risen from 10 to 16 children. The readers had significantly better scores on non-verbal ability, language and short-term memory measures but these could not be demonstrated to be specifically the result of reading progress. However, there was some evidence that early reading skills did predict MLU five years later. The average age of this group was 11 years at the first assessment point and 16 years (range 10 to 24 years) at the second assessment. The actual reading achievements were limited and there is no information on the methods used or time spent on reading activities. It is possible that the gains for spoken language will be seen when teachers are planning to use reading to teach language, and reading activities are engaged in daily. It is also possible that optimal gains for language will be seen when reading is a consistent activity from at least 5 years of age, preferably from 2 to 3 years of age.

In the Byrne (1997) study, all the children were in mainstream placements and there was no significant association between independent reading performance on standardized tests at one phase and language progress at the next phase, to provide specific evidence of reading ability influencing spoken language progress. However, all the children in the Byrne study, regardless of their independent reading ability, were receiving daily reading instruction and inclusion in literacy activities as they recorded their work across the curriculum with support, and the group had significantly better language and short-term memory abilities (Laws, Byrne and Buckley, 2000) and expressive language (Buckley, Sacks, Bird and Archer, 2002) than comparable special school groups. This may suggest that it is the daily involvement in reading experience rather than the child's independent reading skills that leads to gains for spoken language. In the mainstream/special school studies, the comparisons were being made between children who received a high level of reading instruction and literacy experience and those who received very limited literacy instruction or experience of print, if any. More longitudinal research studies are needed to clarify the links between reading and spoken language but, at the present time, the evidence does suggest benefits of reading experience and reading attainments for speech, language and working memory development.

Effective teaching methods that link literacy and speech and language goals

Most authors consider that the principles for teaching children with Down syndrome are the same as for all children (Oelwein, 1995, 1999; Farrell, 1996; Farrell and Gunn, 2000) but teachers should recognize that reading instruction is a very powerful way to teach spoken language and that reading instruction must take account of the child's current language knowledge.

There is no evidence that children with Down syndrome of school age learn to read any differently from other children, but they may rely on a logographic (whole-word) strategy for longer than other children (Byrne, 1997, Kay-Raining Bird, Cleave and McConnell, 2000) and each stage may need to be supported for longer to ensure success. All children use a logographic strategy to read – that is, they memorize the whole word pattern and recognize the word by matching it with their stored word pattern (see Gathercole and Baddeley, 1993a; Oakhill and Beard, 1999; Seymour and Elder, 1986; Seymour, 1993). Children steadily build a store of the visual patterns of written words just as they have built a store of the sound patterns of spoken words, and both these stores are linked to the word meanings (semantic knowledge) and to the grammar (morpho-syntactical knowledge) and speech production (phonological/speech-motor) systems so that they can read words and sentences aloud as well as express their thoughts in spoken words and sentences. Learning about phonics (the link between sounds and letters or letter groups) enables children to develop an alphabetic strategy for decoding and for spelling. Using their letter/sound knowledge, children can sound out the letters when they meet an unfamiliar word and then try to guess the whole word, by *blending* the sounds together, usually using the context of the sentence and text to help them, especially in English, where many word spellings are irregular and cannot be easily decoded (try cough, bough, through, although or yacht, island, knight, laugh). When spelling, the child can think how the word is said, and try to work out the spelling from the sound pattern of the word (this may also need context for clarification – for example 'so', 'sew', 'sow' or 'threw', 'through'). This requires the child to be able to break the sound pattern of the word into component sounds, to *segment* the word. The ability to 'hear' the component sounds in words is called *phonological awareness*. Many typically developing children, who have good spoken language for their age, find this difficult and poor phonological awareness skills are the most common cause of reading difficulties and delays.

There is some evidence that children with Down syndrome do reach a stage when they can use alphabetic strategies for reading and for spelling (Byrne, 1997; Cupples and Iacono, 2000; Kay-Raining Bird, Cleave and McConnell, 2000). Given that most children with Down syndrome have some degree of hearing difficulty and the phonological loop impairment may mean that they are not storing precisely specified and accurate sound patterns for words, it can be predicted that they will have difficulty with phonics and using an alphabetic strategy. Most children and teenagers cannot say all the sounds (phonemes) in the language clearly, adding a further level of difficulty for them. The data collected by Byrne (1997) and Fletcher and Buckley (2002) indicate that children with Down syndrome with mean word reading and spelling ages of about 7 years and above, can use an alphabetic strategy to decode words, and that some are using phonic spelling strategies. Interestingly, the children showed quite good skills in the phonological awareness tasks that required them to detect rhyme, alliteration or to blend, but they found segmenting tasks much more difficult. Alphabetic children, those who could read words they had never seen before because they were artificial or nonsense words made up as an alphabetic test, had good phonological awareness skills, but other children with equally good phonological awareness skills were not yet able to apply them to decoding new words or spelling, highlighting the need to teach these strategies explicitly (Hatcher, Hulme and Ellis, 1994). It takes typically developing children two years to progress from learning the letter-sound links from a phonics teaching programme to being an alphabetic reader and speller in English (see Gathercole and Baddeley, 1993a) suggesting that extensive experience with the printed language is necessary to develop alphabetical skills. Many languages have more regular correspondence between the written and spoken forms of the language than English and these written languages may be easier for children master.

The reader will have noted from the data presented in the first section of this chapter that most children with Down syndrome have word reading and spelling ages ahead of reading comprehension ages. The reasons for this have not been systematically explored. In the studies reported, reading comprehension is usually as good as or better than grammar comprehension. It might be expected that both vocabulary and grammar comprehension levels would predict reading comprehension, and some of the differences (where reading comprehension is ahead of language comprehension) may be an artefact of the different test norms or they may actually demonstrate that some children comprehend written language better than spoken language. More research is needed to explore these relationships. Another factor that can be expected to influence reading comprehension for children with Down syndrome is their limited working memory capacity. It will influence the ability to decode new text while holding in mind the meaning of what has already been read (Gathercole and Pickering, 2000, 2001). Most children with Down syndrome show better comprehension skills when they are reading about activities or characters that are familiar to them, for example reading from their news book, diary or school books when they have recorded information about activities in which they have participated, or reading about familiar television or cartoon characters.

Many children with Down syndrome who can read quite well and read with good comprehension still find writing, in the sense of putting their own thoughts on paper, very difficult and need support to write sentences, short stories or record work. Working memory difficulties will again be part of the explanation as they influence the ability to think what to write next while still recording the previous sentence (Gathercole and Pickering, 2001). Writing difficulties resulting from motor skills delays are a separate issue. Computer software packages may help considerably with both composition and with writing. These include packages that combine symbols with print. The author and colleagues encourage reading instruction using print from the outset rather than symbols, but each child is an individual and symbol systems will help some children to get started, especially if they have experienced reading failure.

Considering the information available, the following principles should inform the teaching of reading to children with Down syndrome:

- start reading activities when child (a) comprehends 50 to 100 spoken words and says or signs some, so is ready to combine words, and (b) can match and select pictures (usually at around 2:6 to 3:6 years of age)
- teach 'sight words' (whole words) first – 'look and say'
- select words as appropriate for the child's language *comprehension* level and interests, starting with words the child already understands
- choose words to make sentences from the start – two key-word and three key-word sentences for children under 4 years but grammatically complete short, simple sentences for all children over 4 years
- make books using pictures of the child's own world and interests to illustrate the sentences
- also play matching and selecting games with the same vocabulary, away from the pictures, to establish confident recognition of the sight vocabulary
- always read the words and sentences with the child while he or she is learning – that is, use errorless learning techniques to prompt success
- from the start ensure that the child understands what he or she is reading – that we read to 'get the message' – just as if someone was talking to us
- once the child is enjoying the reading activities with familiar vocabulary, introduce new vocabulary into the reading
- always encourage the child to repeat the words and sentences with you
- practise writing alongside reading from the start as this will draw attention to letters and help handwriting
- teach phonics once the child has a sight vocabulary of 30 to 40 words (preschoolers) or with the rest of the class – learning to write and spell rhyming sets of words helps phonic skills for all children
- make it fun and recognize that supported reading will develop speech and language skills – the child does not have to be able to read independently for these benefits to occur, although the aim is to have as many children as possible achieve functional literacy skills by their teenage years.

These principles can be applied to beginning readers of any age. Although this chapter has emphasized the importance and particular benefits of introducing reading before 5 years of age, children with Down syndrome may make progress at any age. Teenagers may be motivated to learn to read as they see the practical benefits of learning, and some authors (Fowler, Doherty and Boynton, 1995; Farrell and Elkins, 1991; Farrell, 1996) have emphasized that the cognitive skills of teenagers may mean that they are better able to make progress than in earlier years and that schools should not give up formal literacy teaching in teenage years. An adult literacy programme in Australia is reporting reading progress for young adults with Down syndrome, making use of a variety of whole language approaches to support students in experiencing successful literacy, as well as traditional teaching methods (Van Krayenoord, Moni, Jobling and Ziebarth, 2001; Gallaher, Van Kraayenoord, Jobling and Moni, 2002). This project is also making full use of computer-assisted learning and there is now a wide variety of excellent software to support literacy teaching. The benefits of computer-assisted learning for language and literacy for children with Down syndrome have been demonstrated by Meyers (1988. 1990).

The role of the speech and language therapist in supporting literacy teaching

The speech and language therapist can play an important role in supporting literacy teaching in the classroom and in the preschool years. Most importantly, the therapist can ensure that reading is at an appropriate language level for the child, with vocabulary and sentence structures within the child's comprehension. The therapist can help the teacher or parent construct reading activities to specifically teach new vocabulary and grammar to a child, from preschool and throughout the school years. Moreover, all speech and language targets can be incorporated into reading, spelling and phonics activities.

References

Appleton, M (2000). Reading and its relationship to language development: A comparison of pre-school children with Down syndrome, hearing impairment or typical development. Unpublished MPhil thesis, University of Portsmouth, UK.

Appleton M, Buckley S, MacDonald J (2002) The early reading skills of preschoolers with Down syndrome and their typically developing peers – findings from recent research. Down Syndrome News and Update 2: 9–10.

Appleton M, Buckley S, MacDonald J (in press) A longitudinal comparison of the early reading skills of preschoolers with Down syndrome and their typically developing peers. Down Syndrome Research and Practice.

Bochner S, Outhred L., Pieterse M (2001) A study of functional literacy skills in young adults with Down syndrome. International Journal of Disability, Development and Education 48(1): 67–90.

Bird G, Buckley SJ (2002) Reading and Writing Development for Teenagers with Down Syndrome. Portsmouth: Down Syndrome Educational Trust.

Buckley SJ (1985) Attaining basic educational skills: reading, writing and number. In D Lane, B Stratford (eds) Current Approaches to Down Syndrome. London: Holt Saunders, pp. 315–43.

Buckley SJ (1993) Developing the speech and language skills of teenagers with Down syndrome. Down Syndrome Research and Practice 1(2): 63–71.

Buckley SJ (1995) Improving the expressive language skills of teenagers with Down syndrome. Down Syndrome Research and Practice 3(3): 110–15.

Buckley SJ (2000) Speech and Language Development for Individuals with Down Syndrome – an Overview. Portsmouth: Down Syndrome Educational Trust.

Buckley SJ (2001) Reading and Writing for Individuals with Down Syndrome – an Overview. Portsmouth: Down Syndrome Educational Trust.

Buckley SJ, Bird G (1993) Teaching children with Down syndrome to read. Down Syndrome Research and Practice 1(1): 34–41.

Buckley SJ, Bird G (2001a) Memory Development for Individuals with Down Syndrome. Portsmouth: Down Syndrome Educational Trust.

Buckley SJ, Bird G (2001b) Speech and Language Development for Teenagers with Down Syndrome. Portsmouth: Down Syndrome Educational Trust.

Buckley SJ, Bird G, Byrne A (1996a) Reading acquisition by young children. In B Stratford, P Gunn (eds) New Approaches to Down Syndrome. London, England: Cassell, pp. 268–79.

Buckley SJ, Bird G, Byrne A (1996b) The practical and theoretical significance of teaching literacy skills to children with Down syndrome. In Jean A Rondal and Juan Perera (eds) Down Syndrome: Psychological, Psychobiological and Socio-educational Perspectives. London, England: Whurr, pp. 119–28.

Buckley S, Bird G, Sacks B, Archer T (in press) An evaluation of inclusive and special education for teenagers with Down syndrome: effects on social and academic development. Down Syndrome Research and Practice.

Buckley S, Bird G, Sacks B, Archer T (2002) A comparison of mainstream and special education for teenagers with Down syndrome: implications for parents and teachers. Down Syndrome News and Update 2(2): 46–57.

Buckley SJ, Sacks BI (2002) An overview of the development of teenagers with Down syndrome. Portsmouth; Down Syndrome Educational Trust.

Buckley SJ, Sacks B (1987) The Adolescent with Down Syndrome: Life for the Teenager and for the Family. Portsmouth: University of Portsmouth.

Byrne A (1997) Teaching Reading to Children with Down Syndrome. Unpublished PhD Thesis. University of Portsmouth.

Byrne A, Buckley SJ, MacDonald J, Bird G (1995) Investigating the literacy, language and memory skills of children with Down syndrome and their mainstream peers. Down Syndrome Research and Practice 3(2): 53–8.

Byrne A, MacDonald J, Buckley SJ (2002) Reading, language and memory skills: a comparative longitudinal study of children with Down syndrome and their mainstream peers. British Journal of Educational Psychology.

Carr J, Hewitt S (1982) Children with Down syndrome growing up. Association for Child Psychology and Psychiatry News 10: 10–13.

Chapman RS (1999) Language development in children and adolescents with Down syndrome. In JF Miller, M Leddy, LA Leavitt (eds) Improving the communication of people with Down syndrome. Baltimore Md: Paul H Brookes Publishing Co, pp. 41–60.

Chapman RS, Hesketh LJ (2001) Language, cognition, and short-term memory in individuals with Down syndrome. Down Syndrome Research and Practice 7(1): 1–8.

Cupples L, Iacono T (2000) Phonological awareness is related to reading skill in children with Down syndrome. Journal of Speech, Language and Hearing Research 43: 595–608.

Dickinson LL (2002) The use of a reading programme and signing to develop language and communication skills in a toddler with Down syndrome. Down Syndrome News and Update 2(1): 2–4.

Dodd B, Thompson L (2001) Speech disorder in children with Down's syndrome. Journal of Intellectual Disability Research 45(4): 308–16.

Dykens EM, Hodapp RM, Evans, DW (1994) Profiles and development of adaptive behaviour in children with Down syndrome. American Journal on Mental Retardation 98(5): 580–7.

Duffen L (1976) Teaching reading to children with little or no language. Remedial Education 11(3): 139–42.

Ellis N, Large B (1988) The early stages of reading: a longitudinal study. Applied Cognitive Psychology 2(1): 47–76.

Farrell M (1996) Continuing literacy development. In Brian Stratford, Pat Gunn (eds) New Approaches to Down Syndrome. London: Cassell, pp. 280–99.

Farrell M, Elkins J (1991) Literacy and the adolescent with Down Syndrome. In CJ Denholm, J Ward (eds) Adolescents with Down Syndrome: International Perspectives on Research and Programme Development. Implications for Parents, Researchers and Practitioners. Victoria: University of Victoria, pp. 15–26.

Farrell M, Gunn P (2000) Literacy for Children with Down Syndrome: Early Days. Flaxton, Australia: Post Pressed.

Fletcher H, Buckley SJ (2002) Phonological awareness in children with Down syndrome. Down Syndrome Research and Practice 8(1): 11–18.

Fowler AE, Doherty BJ, Boynton L (1995) The basis of reading skill in young adults with Down syndrome. In Lynn Nadel and Donna Rosenthal (eds) Down Syndrome: Living and Learning in the Community. New York: Wiley Liss, pp. 182–96.

Gallaher KM, Van Kraayenoord CE, Jobling A, Moni KB (2002) Reading with Abby: a case study of individual tutoring with a young adult with Down syndrome. Down Syndrome Research and Practice 8(2): 59–66.

Gathercole SE, Baddeley A (1993a) Working Memory and Language. Hove: Erlbaum.

Gathercole, SE and Baddeley AD (1993b). Phonological working memory: a critical building block for reading development and vocabulary acquisition? European Journal of Psychology of Education 8(3): 259–72.

Gathercole SE, Pickering SJ (2000) Working memory deficits in children with low achievements in the national curriculum at seven years of age. British Journal of Educational Psychology 70(2): 177–94.

Gathercole SE, Pickering SJ (2001) Working memory deficits in children with special educational needs. British Journal of Special Education 28(2): 89–97.

Grove N (1998) Literature for All – Developing. London: David Fulton Publishers.

Hatcher P, Hulme C, Ellis AW (1994) Ameliorating early reading failure by integrating the teaching of reading and phonological skills: the phonological link hypothesis. Child Development 65: 41–57.

Irwin KC (1989) The school achievement of children with Down's syndrome. New Zealand Medical Journal 102(860): 11–13.

Jarrold C, Baddeley AD, Philips C (1999) Down syndrome and the phonological loop: Evidence for, and importance of, a specific verbal short term memory deficit. Down Syndrome Research and Practice 6(2): 61–75.

Jarrold C, Baddeley AD (2001) Short-term memory in Down syndrome: applying the working memory model. Down Syndrome Research and Practice 7(1): 17–23.

Kay-Raining Bird E, Cleave PL, McConnell LM (2000) Reading and phonological awareness in children with Down syndrome: a longitudinal study. American Journal of Speech-Language Pathology 9: 319–30.

Kliewer C (1998) Citizenship in the literate community: an ethnography of children with Down syndrome and the written word. Exceptional Children 64(2): 167–80.

Kotlinski J, Kotlinski S (2002) Teaching reading to develop language. Down Syndrome News and Update 2(1): 5–6.

Laws G, Buckley SJ, Bird G, MacDonald J, Broadley I (1995) The influence of reading instruction on language and memory development in children with Down syndrome. Down Syndrome Research and Practice 3(2): 59–64.

Laws G, Byrne A, Buckley SJ (2000) Language and memory development in children with Down syndrome at mainstream and special schools: a comparison. Educational Psychology 20(4): 447–57.

Laws G, Bishop DVM (2002) A comparison of language impairment in adolescents with Down syndrome and children with specific language impairment. Paper presented at the UK Down Syndrome Research Forum meeting, Portsmouth, May.

Laws G, Gunn D (2001) Relationships between reading, phonological skills and language development in individuals with Down syndrome: a five year follow up study. Reading and Writing 15: 1–22.

Locke JL (1994) Gradual emergence of developmental language disorders. Journal of Speech and Hearing Research 37(3): 608–16.

Locke JL (1997) A theory of neurolinguistic development. Brain and Language 58: 265–326.

Marcell MM (1995) Relationships between hearing and auditory cognition in Down syndrome youth. Down Syndrome Research and Practice 3(3): 373–98.

Mayberry RI, Lock E, Kazmi H (2002) Linguistic ability and early language exposure. Nature 417: 38.

Meyers LF (1988) Using computers to teach children with Down syndrome spoken and written language skills. In Lynn Nadel (ed.) The Psychobiology of Down Syndrome. Cambridge Mass: MIT Press, pp. 247–65.

Meyers LF (1990) Language Development and Intervention. In Don C van Dyke, D Lang, F Heide, S van Duyne, MJ Soucek (eds) Clinical Perspectives in the Management of Down Syndrome. New York NY: Springer-Verlag, pp. 153–64.

Miller JF (1999) Profiles of language development in children with Down syndrome. In JF Miller, M Leddy, LA Leavitt (eds) Improving the communication of people with Down syndrome. Baltimore Md: Paul H Brookes Publishing Co, pp. 41–60.

Oakhill J, Beard R (eds) (1999) Reading Development and the Teaching of Reading: A Psychological Perspective. Oxford: Blackwell Science.

Oelwein PL (1995) Teaching Reading to Children with Down Syndrome: a Guide for Parents and Teachers. Bethesda Md: Woodbine House.

Oelwein PL (1999) Individualizing reading for each child's ability and needs. In Terry J Hassold and David Patterson (eds) Down Syndrome: A Promising Future, Together. New York: Wiley Liss, pp. 155–64.

Oke MK (2002) Teaching Nazli in Turkish and English. Down Syndrome News and Update 2(1): 8.

Pieterse M, Center Y (1984) The integration of eight Down's Syndrome children into regular schools. Australia and New Zealand Journal of Developmental Disabilities 10(1): 20.

Pieterse M (1988) The Down syndrome program at Macquarie University: a model early intervention program. In M Pieterse, S Bochner, S Bettison (eds) Early Intervention for Children with Disabilities: The Australian Experience. Sydney: Macquarie University, pp. 81–96.

Rozen G (2002) Teaching Charlotte spoken language through reading. Down Syndrome News and Update 2(1): 7.

Seymour PHK (1993) A 'dual foundation' model of orthographic development. Presented at Acquisition de la lecture écriture et psychologie cognitive Paris.

Seymour PH, Elder L (1986) Beginning reading without phonology. Cognitive Neuropsychology 3(1): 1–36.

Shott SR (2000) Down syndrome: common paediatric ear, nose and throat problems. Down Syndrome Quarterly 5(2): 1–6.

Stothard SE, Snowling MJ, Bishop DV, Chipchase BB, Kaplan CA (1998) Language impaired preschoolers: a follow up into adolescence. Journal of Speech Language Hearing Research 41(2): 407–18.

Van Kraayenoord CE, Moni KB, Jobling A, Ziebarth K (2001) Broadening approaches to literacy education for young adults with Down syndrome. In M Cuskelly, A Jobling, S Buckley (eds) Down Syndrome across the Life Span. London: Whurr.

Chapter 10
Continued language intervention with adolescents and adults with Down syndrome

CHRISTINE JENKINS

Introduction

In comparison to the research that has been carried out concerning the abilities of children with Down syndrome, the number of studies that have concentrated on adults, or even older adolescents, is very small (Parmenter, 1996). The proportion of this research that has investigated and evaluated the effectiveness of interventions is even smaller. It is not difficult to understand the reason for this. It is in early childhood that most rapid development takes place and at which most intervention has been targeted. Another major influencing factor has been the lifespan of people with Down syndrome. When average life expectancy meant that most people with Down syndrome did not survive adolescence, then studying how people functioned in adult life would not have been a priority. Changes in this area have been dramatic. In 1961 the average life expectancy for people with Down syndrome was 18 years, compared to the present when 70% are expected to live beyond 50 years of age (Oliver and Holland, 1986). This increase has been a mixed blessing, however. It has been accompanied by the development of pre-senile dementia in many older people with Down syndrome.

Intervention to promote the communication of people with Down syndrome when they reach late adolescence and adulthood has had a low profile until recent times. Even now there is a limited amount of work in this area, although there is increasing interest and pressure from families for intervention to continue into adulthood. Medical advances mean the people with Down syndrome have not only a significantly increased life expectancy (Oliver and Holland, 1986) but also better health in their adult years. Parents of adolescents and younger adults have seen the benefits of education and therapy and see no reason why this should stop when their children leave the school system. There are many more opportunities for people with Down syndrome to have a job and play a part in the community, but effective communication is vital to make these opportunities into a reality (Rondal and Comblain, 1996).

The first part of this chapter is concerned with what is known about the language skills of people with Down syndrome when they reach adolescence and adulthood and their abilities in related cognitive and sensory areas, such as hearing. The major issue in researching the abilities of people in this age group with Down syndrome is whether their skills remain stable, continue to develop or decline.

The facility to use language to communicate is an essential part of living an integrated and fulfilling life within the community, but of equal importance is the ability to understand the complexities of what others say (verbal comprehension). The second part of this chapter discusses implications for effective intervention with both expressive language and comprehension. Good language skills alone are not enough. Successful communication involves making the best use of one's skills, whether verbal or non-verbal, and this is discussed together with other significant factors that affect the communication of adults with Down syndrome.

The language skills of adolescents and adults with Down syndrome

Key factors in the discussion of the language skills of people with Down syndrome beyond early adolescence are the role of the critical period, as proposed by Lenneberg (1967) and Fowler's (1990) suggested syntactic ceiling effect.

Critical period hypothesis

Lenneberg (1967) developed the idea of a critical period in development as an explanation for the slowing down of language development in adolescence. He suggested that this is due to loss of brain 'plasticity' at or around puberty. There are examples in the literature of people who for various reasons have not acquired language within the normal developmental period. These examples include Genie, the 'wild child' (Curtiss, 1977) and Chelsea (Curtiss, 1988) who was deaf as a child but became able to hear speech as an adult through amplification. Although vocabulary and basic sentences were acquired, none of these people were able to use complex language structures or learn grammatical rules.

A possible rationale for the limitations of language syntactic development beyond childhood is that the mechanisms controlling phonology and syntax (the 'computational' aspects of language) have specific maturational constraints related to their location in the left hemisphere of the brain. However, the findings of Chua, Weeks and Elliott (1996) that, unlike the general population, speech perception in people with Down syndrome seems to be located in the right hemisphere make the position much more complex. Rondal (1996) did note that he has found a limited improvement in sentence understanding in adults with Down syndrome, but queried whether this is truly evidence of linguistic development or a reflection of improved skills in response to testing. However, he said that 'In contrast to phonology and morpho-syntax, continued improvement beyond childhood seems to be generally the case for referential lexical abilities and pragmatics' (Rondal, 1996: 105).

Chapman (1999), however, found no evidence of a limiting effect of this critical period in her cross-sectional study of children and older teenagers with Down syndrome. She found that MLU increased from an average of 2 for children aged between 5 and 8 years to a mean of 4.3 for those aged from 16 to 20 years. The increase in MLU between the younger and older groups was statistically significant both for narrative and conversation. This study confirmed earlier results from Chapman, Schwartz and Kay-Raining Bird (1992). Chapman attributed some of the earlier findings (for example Fowler, 1990) of a plateau in MLU at adolescence to methodological differences. She emphasized the importance of collecting both narrative and conversational samples, as narrative samples contained consistently longer mean length utterances than conversation.

There is also evidence that teenagers can benefit from language intervention specifically targeted at syntax. Eleven out of 12 young people aged from 13 years 4 months to 15 years 11 months showed an increase in the length and complexity of their sentences following a 12-month intervention (Buckley, 1995). The intervention involved a structured language-teaching programme supported by reading materials. Buckley concluded:

> This study should be seen as encouraging but preliminary. There is an urgent need for speech and language intervention for people with Down's syndrome to be evaluated. Too much of the literature seems to suggest that the usual difficulties are an inevitable consequence of the syndrome, particularly the poor grammar, yet there is no justification for this view until intensive interventions have been thoroughly investigated and evaluated. (Buckley, 1995, p. 115)

There is considerable evidence for a limitation of language development, particularly syntactic skills, to a critical period during childhood. This evidence has a strong theoretical element, supported by practical observations. There is also strong practical evidence that, in people with Down syndrome, syntactic development may continue into adulthood, although structured intervention may be needed to achieve this. This important debate would benefit, as Buckley pointed out, from more research into the language abilities of this age group. Rondal and Comblain (1996) said that a dearth of longitudinal studies makes predictions or assumptions of whether language growth is possible in adulthood difficult. They point to the effect of changes in educational and social circumstances on different age cohorts as a difficulty in cross-sectional studies.

Syntactic ceiling hypothesis

Fowler (1990) proposed the concept of a syntactic ceiling, limiting the language development of people with Down syndrome to simple structures and short sentences. This has similarities to the critical period hypothesis in that it seeks to explain why most people with Down syndrome do not progress beyond a basic linguistic level. However, while the critical period hypothesis places a time limit on development, the syntactic ceiling effect implies a limit in the ability to acquire complex language.

Chapman rejected this theory with evidence from her own research (Chapman, 1999). She found that not only did the length of utterance increase with age but also that the longer sentences were likely to be more complex. Chapman and her colleagues did find that the older group with Down syndrome gave more single-morpheme responses than a control group matched for MLU, but when they analysed the context of these responses found that they 'turned out to be the product of their more advanced comprehension and social understanding' (Chapman, 1999: 51). Their more advanced pragmatic skills meant that they had a better understanding of the questioner's meaning and were able to respond more directly.

Hearing loss in adults with Down syndrome

Comprehensive research studies (Davies, 1996; Marcell and Cohen, 1992; Yeates, 1992) have shown increased likelihood of hearing loss in adolescents and adults with Down syndrome. Moreover, these problems are almost certain to worsen with age. Both conductive and sensory hearing loss is common and many people may experience a combination of both types. In Yeates' study, 64% of the group of adults with Down syndrome was found to have a hearing loss severe enough to warrant amplification. Marcell and Cohen found evidence of high-frequency loss normally associated with ageing (presbyacusis) in a group of older adolescents with Down syndrome with a mean age of 18 years 10 months. It also appeared, from the results of Davies, Yeates, and Marcell and Cohen that, unlike in the general population, where conductive problems usually resolve in early childhood, they frequently persist into adult life for people with Down syndrome.

It is highly likely that such degrees of hearing loss will have an effect on communication skills and it is important to take this into account when considering any type of language intervention.

Implications for language intervention

When we consider language intervention with adolescents and adults with Down syndrome there are two major questions facing us. First, is there any evidence that intervention has any benefits for this age group? Second, what are the most effective ways of delivering such interventions? The dearth of research information relating to language and intervention with people with Down syndrome beyond early adolescence, as discussed in the introduction to this chapter, means that there are no easy answers to either of these questions. It has therefore been reasonable to argue, in the absence of evidence to the contrary, that language intervention for older people with Down syndrome is not an effective use of resources. This can then become a 'self-fulfilling prophesy' – there is no evidence that intervention is effective, therefore little or no intervention takes place, consequently there continues to be no evidence that intervention is effective. However, a small number of studies that have been carried out in recent years do provide some valuable indications concerning effective intervention.

The benefits of language intervention

Research by Buckley (1995), Leddy and Gill (1999) and Jenkins (2001) all provide evidence for the success of language intervention beyond early adolescence. Buckley's study with teenagers and Jenkins' intervention with adults aged between 19 and 49 years both involved structured language teaching targeting the morphosyntactic aspects of expressive language and comprehension. There were significant increases in the use of articles, auxiliary verbs and present and past-tense verb endings, plurals, prepositions and pronouns in both studies. Buckley's study also showed significant increase in the length of sentences. There were similar improvements in comprehension. This is especially relevant for two reasons. Expressive syntax is identified as the most severely affected aspect of language for people with Down syndrome (Miller, 1988) and, according to Rondal (1996), it is the least likely aspect to respond to intervention in adulthood.

Leddy and Gill (1999) were initially sceptical about the possibility of intervening to improve the language skills of adults with Down syndrome. The results of their intervention with five adults caused them to admit 'We were wrong!' (p. 206). They go on to say 'Our sample was small, but each individual was able to achieve a measure of success' (p. 213).

One difference in the findings of Leddy and Gill (1999) and Jenkins (2001) was the effect that age had on the communication skills of the people with Down syndrome. Leddy and Gill, when describing their intervention commented that:

> The older adults who participated in assessments and in therapy did not exhibit the same skills that the younger adults evinced. These older adults did not have functional reading skills. They often would defer to their

caregivers and family members to communicate for them rather than speak for themselves. In addition, these older adults were passive communicators who did not appear to know how to play the communication game. (p. 212)

As Leddy and Gill (1999) did not specify exactly what they mean by 'older' adults it is difficult to make comparisons with any degree of certainty. It is true that none of the participants in Jenkins' (2001) study over 40 years of age had reading skills. On the other hand, they were as eager to communicate and to learn as their younger colleagues. Moreover, Jenkins found no correlation between age and progress on any of the measures used in the study.

Effective intervention strategies

Although the research about effective language intervention with older adolescents and adults with Down syndrome is limited, there is a larger body of evidence concerning the cognitive and language-processing abilities of people with Down syndrome. A number of researchers have found that auditory memory and processing skills are relatively more impaired than skills in the visual domain (Hulme and Mackenzie, 1992; Pueschel, 1988; Marcell and Armstrong, 1982). There is also evidence of successful intervention with children with Down syndrome based on building on strengths in the visual modalities to circumvent some of the weaknesses in auditory processing and memory. Other factors that have proved important in making intervention effective are: structured language teaching, generalizing skills to real-life social interactions and creating communication success.

Visual strategies to support language teaching

There are two specific strategies that have been used to support language teaching and communication in people with Down syndrome: manual signing and the use of reading and writing.

Signing

Signing can be used either as an alternative to spoken language, to augment or supplement speech that is difficult to understand or to facilitate the development of verbal comprehension. It may serve several of these purposes at once in any one individual or it may continue to be used once its original purpose has changed. An older child or adult may have been originally introduced to signing to facilitate language development but may find benefits with continuing to sign to augment their spoken language.

Signing has benefits for both comprehension and expression. Comprehension is made easier because it overcomes many of the auditory memory and processing problems experienced by people with Down syndrome. Romski, Sevcik and Ellis Joyner (1984) suggest that signing may also be less arbitrary than speech. It is true that some signs, usually those expressing abstract concepts, are arbitrary, but many, such as 'drink' or 'house' are closely related to the concepts they represent and, as such, are easier to understand than words. We know that adults with Down syndrome are more likely than not to have some degree of hearing loss (Yeates, 1992) and signing provides an additional channel for receiving language in these circumstances.

Signing can also be used to overcome some of the language production difficulties of people with Down syndrome. Buckley and Bird (1993) observed that young children learning to read would use a sign before saying the word, suggesting that the manual language might act as a bridge to verbal production. Powell and Clibbens (1994) found that when adults with Down syndrome used signing alongside speech, the intelligibility of their speech improved. Signing is a valuable strategy for teaching expressive language skills as it can be used to prompt the production of longer sentences and specific syntactic structures. Unfortunately, as Grove (1993) found, signing may be discontinued once a certain level of language competence is reached. It is important to continue to encourage the use of signing alongside speech. Buckley and Sacks (1987) and Bray and Woolnough (1988) found that signing was an effective repair strategy for the teenagers with Down syndrome in their studies when verbal communication broke down.

Reading

Reading, like signing, at least in its early stages, uses a visual rather than an auditory input channel. It has the advantage over signing and speech of being less transitory. Two studies with older adolescents and adults have built on the work with young children at the beginning of language acquisition (Buckley and Bird, 1993), using reading as a medium for teaching language, specifically the syntactic aspects of language. In Buckley's (1995) study the teenagers who were taught using reading made significantly greater progress on three of the six structures taught than the matched group where spoken language alone was used. Jenkins (2001) did not find the same effect for reading in her study where two matched groups of adults took part in a structured language programme over two years. However, although there were no significant differences between the groups, whether they were taught using reading or spoken language, both groups made significant progress in aspects of morphosyntax with expressive language and comprehension. Comments from the tutors in this study indicated that they found it easier to teach language structures with the aid of the reading materials. Reading may therefore be a useful teaching strategy even though its use did not bring about significantly greater progress. In addition, some of the participants with Down syndrome who were previously nonreaders acquired measurable reading skills during the study. Fowler, Doherty and Boynton (1994) suggest that even a small amount of reading ability may increase self-esteem.

Leddy and Gill (1999) also used reading and writing as a teaching strategy. They found it a useful way to indicate grammatical markers such as 'ed' endings for the past tense, functions words ('a', 'the', and so forth) and to encourage longer sentences. Leddy and Gill describe how Nicholas, a man with Down syndrome, would be helped to record what he wanted to say, using appropriate syntax, on a marker board. Nicholas would then communicate his message, first with the board as a prompt and then without a prompt.

In Jenkins' (2001) intervention, sets of coloured photographs were compiled for each linguistic structure with words, phrases and sentences on separate cards. The teaching objectives for each linguistic structure or concept were:

- recognize and identify materials
- match words to words, phrases to phrases, sentences to sentences
- match words/phrases/sentences to pictures
- identify words/phrases/sentences
- read words/phrases/sentences with picture prompt
- read words/phrases/sentences without picture prompt.

As it increasingly becomes normal practice for children with Down syndrome to learn to read in school (Buckley, Bird and Byrne, 1996) many more will be competent readers by the time they finish full-time education. In these circumstances teaching language, especially the computational aspects of language, through reading is likely to be accepted as an effective and useful strategy. On the other hand, lack of reading skills need not be a barrier to making progress with this method of teaching. Buckley (1993) found that the two teenagers in her study who made the most progress had virtually no reading ability at the start of the programme.

Structured language teaching

As the majority of people with Down syndrome reach adulthood with limited language skills, it is apparent that they have not been able to learn effectively through informal means, as typically developing children do. It is therefore important to use a structured programme of teaching. This comprises assessment to establish an appropriate starting point, a teaching programme based on the sequence of typical language development and setting carefully targeted goals. Leddy and Gill (1999: 207) describe this process in their programme as 'treatment was aimed at achieving a series of small skill goals that would lead to greater success when these goals were combined to achieve larger communication goals.'

Many language-teaching programmes (for example the Derbyshire Language Scheme) (Masidlover and Knowles, 1982) were originally designed for children but can be adapted for use with adults by substituting vocabulary and other content more appropriate for the lives of adults. These adaptations can be used to include materials that relate specifically to the needs and interests of the people involved in the programme, for example using photographs of the people themselves, their friends and families. Using a structured approach enables success to be built into the programme. Research by Wishart (1993) showed that many children with Down syndrome develop strategies for avoiding tasks that they perceive as difficult and become demotivated if the tasks are too easy. Although this research has not been repeated with older adolescents and adults with Down syndrome, it is good practice in teaching and therapy to try to ensure successful outcomes, especially in a group of people who will have experienced at least a measure of communication failure in their lifetimes.

Generalization

Being able to use language with better syntax and sentence length within a structured teaching situation is only part of the process. It is necessary to learn to use these language skills appropriately in everyday social situations. This may not happen spontaneously, and opportunities to practise newly acquired skills should therefore be built into teaching programmes (Leddy and Gill, 1999). Some of this is achieved by ensuring that the teaching objectives will be useful in the individual's daily life. Some people may need the opportunity to practise their new skills in a semi-structured situation. Such practice could include activities such as roleplays, video- or audio-taping conversations and playing them back to enable the individual to monitor his or her own communication skills, or using scripts as prompts.

Communication success

Good language skills are only one part of effective communication, important though they are. Miller (1999: 13) wrote 'Nor does performance at one language level describe an individual's ability to communicate. That is, having a large vocabulary does not automatically mean that the individual can use those words to make sentences or that the sentences the individual uses communicate a message effectively.'

Being a competent communicator also requires the ability to take into account the needs of the listener, or communication partner. It involves strategies to gain attention and establish a topic, turn-taking in conversation and methods for dealing with breakdowns in communication (repair strategies). Most research indicates that people with Down syndrome have good skills in these areas (Miller, 1987). However, two studies concerning the communication skills of teenagers with Down syndrome (Bray and Woolnough, 1988; Buckley and Sacks, 1987) highlighted the need for effective repair strategies. In particular, they identified signing as a means of overcoming either poor intelligibility or limited language skills. Some people with Down syndrome experience frequent breakdowns in communication, often leading to frustration and lack of self-esteem. Signing is not the only strategy that can be useful. Other alternative and augmentative forms of communication such as rebus symbols, pictures or writing can be effective. It is also possible to teach other verbal repair strategies, for example rephrasing the message rather than repeating it.

Conclusions

Although research concerning effective language intervention with adolescents and adults with Down syndrome is limited at this time, there is sufficient evidence to give indications for good practice. These include:

- building on strengths in the visual domain to support language teaching, in particular using signing, reading and writing
- using structured language programmes with easily achievable, specific goals linked to the interests and communication needs of the participants
- including opportunities for generalizing newly acquired skills to everyday social situations
- creating communication success by teaching strategies to cope with communication breakdowns.

There is growing evidence that language intervention can be successful for people with Down syndrome in adult life. There is likely to be increasing pressure from families and carers and people with Down syndrome themselves for intervention and therapy to continue beyond childhood. According to Leddy and Gill (1999: 213) 'The future for adults with Down syndrome is promising.' It is the responsibility of researchers, service providers and individual professionals to ensure that the promise becomes a reality.

References

Bray M, Woolnough L (1988) The language skills of children with Down's syndrome aged 12 to 16 years. Child Language Teaching and Therapy 4(3): 311–24.

Buckley S (1993) Developing the speech and language skills of teenagers with Down's syndrome. Down's Syndrome: Research and Practice 1(2): 63–71.

Buckley S (1995) Improving the expressive language skills of teenagers with Down's syndrome. Down's Syndrome: Research and Practice 3(3): 110–15.

Buckley S, Bird G, Byrne A (1996) Reading acquisition by young children with Down's syndrome. In B Stratford, P Gunn (eds) New Approaches to Down Syndrome. London: Cassell, pp. 268–79.

Buckley S, Bird G (1993) Teaching young children with Down's syndrome to read. Down's Syndrome: Research and Practice 1(1): 34–8.

Buckley S, Sacks B (1987) The adolescent with Down's syndrome. Portsmouth: Portsmouth Down's Syndrome Trust.

Chapman R (1999) Language development in children and adolescents with Down syndrome. In JF Miller, M Leddy, LA Leavitt (eds) Improving the communication of people with Down syndrome. Baltimore: Paul H Brookes, pp. 41–60.

Chapman R, Schwartz S, Kay-Raining Bird E (1992) Language production of older children with Down syndrome. 9th World Congress of the International Association for the Scientific Study of Mental Deficiency.

Chua R, Weeks D, Elliott D (1996) A functional systems approach to understanding verbal-motor integration in individuals with Down's syndrome. Down's Syndrome: Research and Practice 4(1): 25–36.

Curtiss S (1977) Genie: a psycholinguistic study of a modern-day 'wild child'. New York: Academic Press.

Curtiss S (1988) The special talent of grammar acquisition. In L Obler, D Fein (eds) The Exceptional Brain. New York: Guilford, pp. 364–86.

Davies B (1996) Auditory disorders. In B Stratford, P Gunn (eds) New Approaches to Down Syndrome. London: Cassell, pp. 100–21.

Fowler A (1990) Language Abilities in Children with Down Syndrome: Evidence for a Specific Syntactic Delay. In D Cicchetti, M Beeghly (eds) Children with Down syndrome: A Developmental Perspective. New York: Cambridge University Press, pp. 302–28.

Fowler A, Doherty B, Boynton L (1994) The basis of reading skills in young adults with Down syndrome. In D Rosenthal, L Nadel (eds) Down Syndrome: Living and Learning in the Community. New York: Wiley-Liss, pp. 182–96.

Grove N (1993) Good with their Hands? Analysing the Skills of Signers with Learning Disabilities. Child Language Seminar, Plymouth.

Hulme C, Mackenzie S (1992) Working Memory and Severe Learning Difficulties. Hove: Lawrence Erlbaum Associates.

Jenkins C (2001) Adults with Down syndrome: an investigation of the effect of reading on language skills. Unpublished Doctoral Thesis. Portsmouth: University of Portsmouth.

Leddy M, Gill G (1999) Enhancing the speech and language skills of adults with Down syndrome. In JF Miller, M Leddy, LA Leavitt (eds) Improving the Communication of People with Down Syndrome. Baltimore: Paul H Brookes, pp. 205–13.

Lenneberg E (1967) Biological Foundations of Language. New York: Wiley.

Marcell M, Armstrong V (1982) Auditory and visual sequential memory of Down's syndrome and non-retarded children. American Journal of Mental Deficiency 87(1): 86–95.

Marcell M, Cohen S (1992) Hearing abilities of Down syndrome and other mentally handicapped adolescents. Research in Developmental Disabilities 13(6): 533–51.

Masidlover M, Knowles W (1982) The Derbyshire Language Scheme. Alfreton: Derbyshire County Council.

Miller JF (1988) The developmental asynchrony of language development in Down syndrome. In L Nadel (ed.) The Psychobiology of Down's Syndrome. New York: NDSS, pp. 167–98.

Miller JF (1987) Language and communication characteristics of children with Down syndrome. In S Pueschel, C Tingey, J Rynders, A Crocker, D Crutcher (eds) New Perspectives on Down Syndrome, Baltimore Md: Paul H Brookes, pp. 233–62.

Miller JF (1999) Profiles of language development in children with Down syndrome. In JF Miller, M Leddy, LA Leavitt (eds) Improving the Communication of People with Down Syndrome. Baltimore Md: Paul H Brookes, pp. 119–32.

Oliver C, Holland A (1986) Down's Syndrome and Alzheimer's Disease: A Review. Psychological Medicine 16: 307–22.

Parmenter TR (1996) Living in the community. In B Stratford, P Gunn (eds) New Approaches to Down Syndrome. London: Cassell, pp. 421–3.

Powell G, Clibbens J (1994) Actions speak louder than words: signing and speech intelligibility in adults with Down's syndrome. Down's Syndrome: Research and Practice 2(3): 127–9.

Pueschel S (1988) Visual and auditory processing in children with Down syndrome. In L Nadel (ed.) The Psychobiology of Down's Syndrome. New York: NDSS, pp. 199–216.

Romski M, Sevcik R, Ellis Joyner S (1984) Non-speech communication systems: implications for intervention with mentally retarded children. Topics in Language Disorder (December): pp. 169–71.

Rondal J (1996) Oral language in Down's syndrome. In J Rondal, J Perera, L Nadel, A Comblain (eds) Down's syndrome. psychological, psychobiological and socio-educational perspectives. London: Whurr, pp. 99–117.

Rondal J, Comblain A (1996) Language in adults with Down's syndrome. Down's Syndrome: Research and Practice 4(1): 3–14.

Wishart J (1993) Learning the hard way: avoidance strategies in young children with Down's syndrome. Down's Syndrome: Research and Practice 1(2): 47–55.

Yeates S (1992) Have they got a hearing loss? Mental Handicap 20: 236–33.

Chapter 11
Maintenance training in older ages[1]

JEAN A RONDAL

Introduction

People with Down syndrome live markedly longer these days than was the case in the last century and before. According to Baird and Sadovnick (1995; data confirmed in other studies regarding various countries such as Dupont, Vaeth and Videbech, 1986; Jancar and Jancar, 1996), estimates predict a life expectancy beyond 68 years for over 15% and 55 years for over 50% of individuals with Down syndrome. Strauss and Eyman (1996) estimate the life expectancy in people with Down syndrome to be around 55 years on average. Further progress may probably still be expected.

These gains in longevity have brought about increased interest in the adult and ageing years of persons with Down syndrome. About three decades ago, however, the possibility of a marked susceptibility of individuals with Down syndrome to a degenerative condition known as Alzheimer disease was identified, as well as a tendency towards earlier anatomo-physiological and neuropsychological ageing when compared with members of the typically ageing population and individuals with an intellectual impairment of other etiologies. It was suggested in some publications that beyond 35 to 40 years most, if not all, persons with Down syndrome would develop a form of Alzheimer disease, leading to major debilitation and the loss of most of the skills acquired earlier in life.

More recent work has softened this dark prognosis. It is admitted now (see, for example, Wisniewski and Silverman, 1999) that trisomy 21 (T21) does not necessarily carry an unavoidable destiny of progressive deterioration during middle age. There is no question, however, that there exists an elevated risk of Alzheimer disease or Alzheimer-like disease (Alzheimer disease actually is not a single disease but a complex of related diseases) in Down syndrome (between 25% and 45% beyond 55 years, according to

166

Zigman, Schup, Haaveman and Silverman, 1997; 19% before and 42% beyond 50 years in Van Buggenhout et al.'s cohort, 2001).

Neurological examination of the brains of persons with Down syndrome who died over the age of 30 years reveal that pathological changes associated with Alzheimer disease (such as brain atrophy, nerve cell loss, neurotransmitter changes, senile plaques, and neurofibrillary tangles – Mann, 1992) have taken place in the amygdala, hippocampus, and the frontal, temporal, and parietal cortices (cf. Holland and Oliver, 1996, for a review). However, for those people with Down syndrome who do develop Alzheimer disease, there is most often a long latency period (in contrast to the usual four or five latency years for the typically ageing population) between the presence of important Alzheimer disease-type neuro-pathological changes and clinical dementia (Wisniewski and Silverman, 1996).

A limited number of studies have centred on cerebral metabolism in older individuals with Down syndrome. Schapiro et al. (1987) measured the cerebral metabolic rate for glucose (CMRG; 18F2 -fluoro-2 deoxydextroglucose) in cohorts of individuals from the typically ageing population and individuals with Down syndrome, aged between 19 and 64 years. Mean hemispheric CMRG was lower in the older than in the younger individuals with Down syndrome (and, as a rule, lower in those with Down syndrome than those in the typically ageing population). Only some older individuals with Down syndrome were clinically demented even if age reductions in neurological variables seemed to occur in most of them. In another cerebral study, however, Schapiro Haxby and Grady (1992) found similar CMRG in non-demented individuals with Down syndrome over 35 years of age and in a typically ageing comparison group. A similar result was reported by Dani et al. (1996). In contrast, Deb, De Silva, Gemmel, Besson, Smith and Ebmeier (1992) reported cerebral metabolic rates in seven older persons with Down syndrome comparable to those of younger people with Down syndrome and slightly diminished rates (particularly in the posterior parietotemporal and occipital zones) in nine other non-demented older people with Down syndrome.

The above statistics and neuropathological indications must be put in context. Developments in the histopathological approach to dementia suggest that age is probably not the sole cause and may not even be the primary cause of senile dementia (Brion and Plas, 1987). A particularly important factor for people with Down syndrome, who are often exposed to less stimulating environment later in life, is that ageing individuals may suffer from (treatable) pseudodementias (sometimes misdiagnosed as depressive states) (see also Campbell-Taylor, 1993; Florez, 2000).

There is, however, an earlier onset of neuropsychological decline in adults with Down syndrome, unrelated to incipient Alzheimer disease for most individuals (Brown, 1985), but more marked than in individuals with intellectual disabilities of etiologies other than Down syndrome

(Thompson, 1999). Van Buggenhout et al. (2001) report a significant increase in the proportions of people with Down syndrome presenting additional health problems beyond 50 years (for example, hearing and sight losses, epilepsy, and hypothyroidy).

Predispositions towards earlier ageing in Down syndrome may be associated with overexpression of genes located on chromosome 21, distinct from the gene coding for amyloid preprotein (residing in the proximal part of the long arm of chromosome 21 and supplying one key factor to Alzheimer disease neuropathology). Similarly, the clinical phenotype of Down syndrome can be modulated by genes on chromosomes other than chromosome 21 (Royston, Mann, Pickering-Brown and Owen, 1994). But these genes remain to be identified (Wisniewski and Silverman, 1996). Research is needed to assess the abilities of individuals with Down syndrome in their 40s, 50s and beyond, and to measure precisely the possible declines in neuropsychological functioning.

Language evolution in adults with Down syndrome

Few specific data have been published so far regarding the language evolution of ageing individuals with Down syndrome. My co-workers and I have collected several series of data relevant to this question (Comblain, 1996; Rondal and Comblain, 1996, 2002; George, Thewis, Van der Linden, Salmon and Rondal, 2001). The same instrument for analysing morphosyntactic aspects of language – the Batterie pour l'Evaluation de la Morpho-Syntaxe (BEMS) (Comblain, 1995) – was used with cohorts of individuals with Down syndrome of different chronological ages (CA) allowing fine cross-sectional comparisons. Each group included seven people (females and males). They were compared on the receptive subtests of the BEMS: nominal co-reference in the case of personal pronouns, definite and indefinite articles, temporal morphological inflections, negative sentences, reversible and nonreversible passive sentences, sentences with coordinate clauses, sentences with temporal, causal, conditional, or consequential subordinate clauses, and sentences with relative subordinates in 'qui' (grammatical subject) or 'que' (direct grammatical object). Table 11.1 lists the definitional characteristics of the three CA samples of persons with Down syndrome (Comparison I). Table 11.2 displays the group means and standard deviations for the eight subtests of the BEMS.

A one-way MANOVA for nonrepeated measures, carried out simultaneously on the eight dependent variables for the three CA groups, revealed no significant statistical difference (at the conventional $p < 0.05$ level) in the receptive morphosyntactic functioning of individuals with Down syndrome from adolescence to mature adulthood over an interval of 32 years. Regarding language production, no direct comparison of the younger and the older adults was possible because, this time, the same set of language productive measures was not used for comparing the adolescent and the younger adult groups (in what were actually two studies) (see Comparison

Table 11.1. Definitional characteristics of the samples of people with Down syndrome (comparison I).

	Adolescents (n=7)	Younger adults (n=7)	Older adults (n=7)
CA[1]			
Mean	16 years 7 months	26 years 9 months	44 years
SD[2]	22 months	32 months	38 months
VI[3]	14 years 5 months–	23 years 4 months–	40 years 5 months–
	19 years 6 months	30 years 1 month	46 years 7 months
MA[4]			
Mean	4 years 4 months	4 years 7 months	4 years 4 months
SD	8 months	9 months	6 months
VI	3 years 8 months–	3 years 6 months–	3 years 9 months–
	5 years 6 months	5 years 3 months	5 years 4 months

Notes: 1. CA: chronological age; 2. SD: standard deviation on the mean; 3. VI: variation interval around the mean; 4. MA: mental age. The differences between mean MAs across CA groups were not statistically significant (one-way ANOVA for unrelated samples).

Table 11.2. Group means and standard deviations from the BEMS subtests in three samples of people with Down syndrome (comparison I).[1]

	People with Down syndrome		
BEMS subtests	Adolescents	Younger adults	Older adults
1. Nominal coreference	43 (8)	48 (35)	51 (15)
2. Articles	30 (6)	34 (8)	36 (17)
3. Temporal inflections	40 (4)	43 (6)	40 (15)
4. Negatives	57 (24)	38 (37)	36 (35)
5. Passives	57 (17)	48 (42)	52 (29)
6. Coordinates	64 (13)	70 (7)	64 (27)
7. Subordinates	43 (21)	31 (25)	51 (20)
8. Relatives	77 (20)	71 (25)	73 (18).

Note. 1. Data are expressed as percentages of correct responses. Standard deviations are given in parentheses.

II below for the productive measures used). The paper by Rondal and Comblain (1996) contains the productive data resulting from the comparison of the same adolescents and younger adults with Down syndrome as in the present report. Accordingly, no significant change was observed as to mean length of utterance (MLU) – a valid if global index of expressive morphosyntax, as is known – and expressive referential lexicon (TVAP: Test de Vocabulaire Actif et Passif; TVP: Test de Vocabulaire Productif). Although we do not have specific data at hand to support our conclusion, it is unlikely that marked changes in productive language take place in the interval of time between 30 and 40 years in people with Down syndrome, particularly given that no significant change has been documented in the receptive abilities of the same people and that no significant productive or receptive change has been revealed either by our analyses of the language of individuals with Down syndrome between 40 and 50 years (see below).

As we indicated a few years ago upon reviewing the specialized literature (cf. Rondal and Comblain, 1996), significant language progress does
not seem to take place, at least in the phonological and the grammatical
aspects, beyond mid-adolescence. As we noted also, progress may still be
observed beyond that age in the conceptual and the pragmatic aspects of
language (for example, vocabulary, conversational and more generally
communicative abilities, and discourse organization; see, for example,
Chapman, 1999, and Berry, Groenweg, Gibson and Brown, 1984). In the
future it will be important to distinguish between the different components of language when considering progress beyond adolescence and to
avoid global maturational hypotheses of the type proposed by Lenneberg
(1967) and Fowler (1990). They suggest that no marked language
improvement at all is possible beyond early adolescence. Lenneberg and
Fowler's characterizations may indeed not be appropriate. The generic
use of the word 'language' provides a problem in their statements. Rondal
and Edwards (1997) have suggested that it makes more theoretical and
empirical sense to restrict the maturational susceptibility to the formal
components of language – phonology and grammar.

We also conducted a four-year longitudinal study with 12 individuals
with Down syndrome aged between 37 and 49 years (6 women and 6
men). Their language functions (receptive as well as productive) were
assessed for every subject at one-year intervals during the first two years.
Four subjects did not maintain their participation beyond the second
year. For the others, the study was continued for another two years using
the same evaluation procedure. For eight individuals (four women and
four men) a measure of cerebral metabolism rate (CMR) for fluoro-
deoxyglucose (18FDG) was made every year using the positron emission
tomography (PET) scan technique and yielding 31 reconstructed plans
from the emission scans (cf. George et al., 2001, for more technical
details). For seven of these eight people (one died in the meantime) the
cerebral imagery investigation was prolonged for two more years with
one examination taking place every year.

Table 11.3 displays the group means and standard deviations resulting
from the analyses of the language of the seven adults with Down syndrome. The BEMS was used to assess receptive morphosyntax. A receptive
lexical task (picture designation) adapted and modified after the test of
Bishop and Byng (1984) was also given. To assess production, a task of verbal (semantic) fluency was used. The adults with Down syndrome were
requested to supply orally the largest possible number of animal names in
one minute. A specially devised test of lexical labelling (picture denomination) was administered. It counted 127 items divided into five semantic
categories (fruits, clothes, vegetables, kitchen tools and objects, and animals). The phonetic length of the items was controlled (items of one, two
or three syllables were presented) as well as the frequency of appearance
of these items in the language (frequency tables for the French language).

Table 11.3. Group means and standard deviations from the receptive and the productive tasks in older adults with Down syndrome at one-year intervals during four years (comparison 2)[1].

Receptive tasks	People with Down syndrome/time			
	1	2	3	4
BEMS				
1. Nominal coreference	51 (15)	29 (9)	39 (17)	40 (15)
2. Articles	36 (17)	23 (7)	27 (11)	28 (16)
3. Temporal inflections	40 (15)	35 (8)	32 (10)	34 (7)
4. Negatives	36 (35)	45 (35)	34 (29)	30 (20)
5. Passives	52 (29)	48 (18)	43 (10)	36 (21)
6. Coordinates	64 (27)	48 (26)	50 (13)	57 (10)
7. Subordinates	51 (20)	47 (14)	39 (13)	37 (15)
8. Relatives	73 (18)	68 (10)	55 (12)	46 (14)
Lexical designation[2]	19 (5)	18 (5)	19 (5)	20 (5)
Productive tasks				
Verbal fluency	10 (5)	9 (4)	8 (3)	8 (3)
Lexical labelling				
TOTAL[3]	144 (17)	137 (33)	135 (28)	137 (33)
Fruits	25 (6)	24 (4)	23 (5)	25 (9)
Clothes	28 (5)	26 (5)	28 (4)	27 (6)
Vegetables	25 (11)	24 (8)	21 (8)	21 (6)
Kitchen tools and objects	33 (4)	31 (8)	30 (8)	32 (6)
Animals	33 (9)	31 (12)	33 (10)	31 (11)
Narrative text about pictures (verbal recall)				
Ideas[4]	3 (1)	3 (1)	2 (2)	3 (2)
Words[5]	10 (4)	10 (6)	7 (5)	8 (6)
Report (morpho-syntactic and semantic aspects)[6]	25 (13)	28 (15)	28 (20)	23 (13)

Notes.
1. BEMS data are expressed as percentages of correct responses. Other data are raw scores of correct responses. Standard deviations are given in parentheses.
2. Maximum correct score is 40.
3. Maximum correct score is 254; maximum correct scores for the semantic categories: fruits, 56, clothes, 48, vegetables, 46, kitchen tools and objects, 52, and animals, 52.
4. Each global idea from the original story correctly recalled was worth 0.5.
5. Number of words per utterance in the story recall; 6. Global index integrating separate scores for the use of causal relations, anaphoric pronouns replacing thematic nouns functioning as sentence subjects, the correct working of chronology in the story, the production of complex sentences, and the number of tenses used in the story recall (maximum note 100).

The participants were allowed 20 seconds for answering. After this time, a phonemic prompt was given (the first phoneme of the target word was supplied by the examiner). In case of further error or absence of response, a syllabic help was given (the first syllable of the target word was produced by the examiner). The aim was to separate a possible lack of the word from a genuine ignorance of the target name. Lastly, the test 'récit sur images' (narrative text about pictures; verbal recall; adapted from Chevrie-Müller, 1981) was administered. This test takes into account the number of global ideas, words, and several formal and semantic characteristics of the narratives as they are freely recalled by the participants.

The one-way (four age levels) multiple analyses of variance (MANOVA) on the eight dependent variables from the BEMS, the analyses of variance (ANOVA) on the lexical designation scores, the ANOVA on the verbal fluency data, MANOVA on the five dependent variables of the test of lexical labelling, and the ANOVA on the total denomination scores failed to yield a significant result, failing therefore to corroborate the null hypothesis of a language change in the adults with Down syndrome across the four-year study.

Turning to the CMR data, the left and right frontal, parietal, and temporal cortices of each adult were examined and the visual metabolic images from the associative cortical regions were evaluated in a semi-quantitative way on a scale from zero (normal metabolism) to two (severe metabolic reduction) (Hoffman et al., 1996; Pickut et al., 1997). As expected, no CMR image proved normal, in the strict interpretation, in any adult with Down syndrome and there was important interindividual variability. Globally, metabolic reduction was more marked at the level of the left hemisphere. Along the time dimension, there was a gradual decrease in global CMR for each of the two cerebral hemispheres and for each of the seven people with Down syndrome (average global CMR for the right hemisphere at times 1 and 3, respectively 1.57 and 3.58; average global CMR for the left hemisphere at times 1 and 3, respectively 2.50 and 5.50). The average decreases, however, were largely due to three participants. Analysing the performance of these three adults in the language tasks over the same interval of time, no evidence of deterioration emerged that could meaningfully be related to the lowering in CMR. It is possible that global brain metabolism (particularly within the left cerebral hemisphere) is diminished substantially in some individuals with Down syndrome without any clear negative consequence on language functioning.

As our series of data show, no major change takes place in the language of individuals with Down syndrome in the interval of time between late adolescence and 50 years. This is worth noting, as functional modifications of language and memory have often been indicated as first signs of earlier ageing and degenerative diseases. Jodar (1992), for example, suggested that in normal ageing, lexical and verbal comprehension in general are preserved whereas verbal fluency, lexical labelling and, more generally, the capacity for verbal production tend to decline. In a cross-sectional work with 44 Italian individuals with Down syndrome (25 males and 19 females) ranging in age from 14 to 43 years and 7 months (average CA 26 years 9 months), which centred on an investigation of the visual-perceptual abilities using the Frostig Developmental Test of Visual Perception (DTVP) (Frostig, Maslow, Lefever and Whittlesy, 1963) and adaptive behaviour using an Italian adaptation (Pedrabissi and Soresi, 1989) of the Adaptive Behaviour Inventory of Brown and Leigh, Saviolo-Negrin, Soresi, Baccichetti, Pozzan and Trevisan (1990) reported no significant age difference in their participants with Down syndrome regarding adaptive behaviour but a significant, even if limited, decline in visual perception beyond 25 years of age, except in the visual-motor sub-test of the DTVP.

What may happen beyond 50 years or so in people with Down syndrome is not predictable at present for lack of systematic data. Hints may be derived from the limited literature in existence, pending verification through more extensive studies. A study by Das, Divis, Alexander, Parrila, and Naglieri (1995) suggests that little or no change in nonverbal reasoning, memory, language (receptive and expressive vocabulary), planning and attention, perceptual-motor, and adaptive skills, occurs until close to 60 years. However, the same authors signal that the older adults with Down syndrome in their cohorts (those slightly beyond 60 years) were actually performing worse than those in younger groups, particularly in tasks requiring planning and attention. This could perhaps be considered in the context of Ribes and Sanuy (2000)'s observation of a slight decline in expressive language (particularly vocabulary) in some of their participants with Down syndrome beyond 38 years, and with Prasher's (1996) suggestion regarding the existence of an age-associated functional decline in short-term memory, speech, practical skills, activity and general interests in approximately 20% of persons with Down syndrome aged 50 to 71 years.

Cross-sectional studies, of course, are limited in their ability (validity) to demonstrate time changes as they compare different individuals at different ages, mixing together interindividual and age-related variances. When considering individuals with Down syndrome the problem is further complicated by a cohort difference: younger persons with Down syndrome have generally been the targets of early cognitive intervention (at least in the developed countries) whereas older individuals with Down syndrome have not had the same input, or only to a lesser extent in the favourable cases. It could be hypothesized that early intervention has the potential effect of upgrading development in many Down syndrome subjects therefore rendering the comparisons with older cohorts of people with Down syndrome difficult or even invalid. A few longitudinal studies have been conducted. Devenny, Hill, Patxot, Silverman and Wisniewski (1992) and Burt, Loveland, Chen, Chuang, Lewis and Cherry (1995) did not observe significant changes in the cognitive functioning of individuals with Down syndrome aged between 27 and 55 years and 22 and 56 years in the two studies, respectively, over intervals of time going from three to five years. Devenny, Silverman, Hill, Jenkins, Sersen and Wisniewski

(1996) report only four cases of cognitive decline in 91 adults with Down syndrome followed for several years beyond the age of 50 years.

The above observations do not suggest rapid and marked age-related decline in the cognitive and language functioning of adults with Down syndrome beyond 50 years, apart from the episodic occurrence of progressive dementia. It may be, however, that, at least for some individuals, a slow gradual language deterioration could be taking place after 50 or 55 years.

An interesting piece of research has come to my attention that may throw further light on the preceding discussion. In 1992 I found myself in a position to analyse the language and cognitive level of a woman named Françoise with Down syndrome. She presented exceptional language abilities for a person with Down syndrome (cf. Rondal, 1995 for the complete report). Recently, the day centre where Françoise (now aged 46) spends several days a week requested a neuropsychological examination motivated by her depressed behaviour, lack of initiative and possible memory losses. Dr Michel Ylieff, a neuropsychologist from the University of Liège who has specialized in the clinical psychological aspects of ageing, carried out a re-examination of some of Françoise's cognitive functions. Comparing his data with those of Rondal (1995), Ylieff (personal communication, May 2000b) signals a marked lowering of Françoise's episodic memory and ability to deal with visuo-spatial and graphic material. Pending further neurological and neuro-radiological examinations, Ylieff suggests a localized pathology of the right cerebral hemisphere possibly linked with incipient brain degeneration. In the last case, the first clinical expression of the neuropathology would be affecting the cognitive domains less well developed – in the case of Françoise, the spatial functions. Regarding oral language, one labelling test yielded a global score closely corresponding to the estimated typical population mean. No morphosyntactic evaluation was attempted. However, based on the three personal encounters with Françoise needed to complete the testing and including informal conversations, Ylieff's impression (Ylieff, 2000b) was that Françoise's overall language was intact as much as could be ascertained, and this was also the opinion of the staff of the day centre attended by Françoise. At age 46, therefore, no major lowering in Françoise's functional language was evident, even if she was experiencing additional difficulties in already weaker other mental functions as a consequence of a possible accelerating ageing or degenerative process.

Language maintenance in later years

The above observations suggest an interesting working hypothesis regarding the onset of mental deterioration in ageing people with Down syndrome. At the individual level, more developed mental functions may resist the degenerative process or the push towards earlier ageing better and for longer for reasons not known at the present time but which might have to do with their relative overrepresentation in the brain circuitry. On the other hand, less developed functions or learned processes would be more vulnerable to incipient degeneration or early ageing. Here, one may repeat the emphasis on the importance of early and continued remedial intervention as a way not only to promote development and better functioning in persons with Down syndrome but also to prepare for better resistance to a possible later life negative change in this syndrome. There is also a slight indication that, as could have been expected, the efficiency of the cognitive programmes is better for those ageing subjects characterized by higher levels of performance prior to training (cf. Aufray and Jukel's 2001 work with typically ageing 80-year-olds). This suggests the importance of finely assessing the relative strengths and weaknesses of ageing people with Down syndrome in order to plan and focus the remedial and maintenance activities most efficiently.

For those individuals with Down syndrome developing Alzheimer disease, the exact pattern of language decline has not been specified yet. In non-disabled individuals, the language changes are most apparent first at the semantic level, particularly in the reduction of available vocabulary and breakdown of semantic associations (Martin, 1987). Difficulty in word finding is one of the most noticeable features of incipient Alzheimer disease. There are also deficits in auditory comprehension of words, as well as in the processing of semantic complexity in sentences and paragraphs (Hart, 1988). Additionally, the quality of discourse, its cohesion, and, in short, the whole pragmatics of language, deteriorates (Maxim and Bryan, 1994).

It is repeatedly observed that the grammatical aspects of language are largely spared in the early stages of Alzheimer disease (Appel, Kertesz, and Fishman, 1982; Kempler, Curtiss, and Jackson, 1987; Murillo Ruiz, 1999). Grammar is eventually disturbed together with the progressive breakdown of the conceptual aspects of language and the collapse of the pragmatic regulations (Maxim and Bryan, 1994).

There is no logical reason why the language fate of individuals with Down syndrome and Alzheimer disease should be any different in basic terms from that of previously non-disabled people. Accordingly, predicted language profiles associated with Alzheimer disease for persons with Down syndrome in the first stages of the disease would be characterized by major dissociations between morphosyntactic, on the one hand, and the semantic and pragmatic aspects of language, on the other hand. The former aspects are underdeveloped in most individuals with Down syndrome. They would be little touched as a direct result of incipient Alzheimer disease. The latter language aspects will be found deteriorating to an extent varying between individuals with Down syndrome.

In people with Down syndrome a marked susceptibility for ageing (biologically as well as neuropsychologically) one or two decades more quickly than non-Down syndrome individuals seems to exist (Vicari, Nocentini and Caltagirone, 1994). The exact causes of this earlier ageing are not known. They may be genetic. The same decline as in healthy older non-disabled people could be the rule for adults with Down syndrome but the decline manifests itself earlier in life. The most frequent speech and language problems encountered in later life by typically ageing individuals are listed in Table 11.4.

Table 11.4. Frequent speech and language difficulties in ageing people (after Rondal and Edwards, 1997).

1. Slower receptive and productive language processing.
2. Less efficient respiratory support for speech.
3. Aggravated hearing problems and reduced attention to auditory stimuli; difficulties in perceiving low-voiced and whispered speech, speech in noisy conditions, and in communicating on the telephone.
4. Additional difficulties in linguistic analysis, particularly with less frequent and longer or more complex syntactic structures.
5. Additional difficulties in planning, producing or monitoring information in spoken discourse.
6. Augmented rates of dysfluencies (hesitation pauses, fillers, and interjections).
7. Reduced word fluency.
8. Increased difficulty in oral word discrimination, and in retrieving infrequently used common and (even more) proper nouns.

Language therapy, or language maintenance, with the typical elderly (for example, Maxim and Bryan, 1994) could be adapted to ageing people with Down syndrome taking into account the particular limitations intrinsic to the condition and already present well before the onset of any ageing or degeneration episode. It could help to reduce their increasing processing difficulties and prevent or delay, to some extent (impossible to define at the present time), the process of decline. Of course, additional studies (particularly longitudinal ones) and more detailed descriptions of language (and cognition) in ageing individuals with Down syndrome are needed before a clearer picture can emerge and a comprehensive theoretical framework be worked out. In the meantime, however, one may usefully propose a series of activities with the general objective of trying to maintain as far as possible the levels of language functioning that have already been attained over many years, no matter how modest they might be. Moreover, the social environments of ageing people with Down syndrome can and should be organized taking the increasing language and cognitive limitations of these people into account. How can this be done? In fact, relatively simple adaptations such as speaking more slowly and slightly more loudly, using shorter and formally simpler utterances, reducing the effects of background noise, allowing additional time for processing incoming language and responding, and arranging settings, seating and lighting to encourage social proximity rather than to limit it, would greatly alleviate the communicative burden of the ageing person with Down syndrome.

How can we envisage and programme language maintenance in ageing persons with Down syndrome? I believe that we should focus, in the first place, on the following items, which I shall develop to some extent: sensitivity to auditory stimuli in various environmental conditions; productive lexical support; receptive and productive language processing and discourse planning and monitoring.

Attending to and discriminating auditory stimuli

Changes in sensory systems (particularly regarding hearing and vision) are a characteristic feature of ageing people with Down syndrome. Some visual deficits tied to ageing (such as cataracts) can be addressed surgically and, evidently, there is no reason to prevent elderly individuals with Down syndrome from accessing these medical possibilities. Additional hearing problems in older people may be more difficult to identify because they are more diffuse. Often they are accompanied by a weakening of attention (and perhaps interest) towards auditory stimuli, particularly in the speech and musical sound frequencies (roughly between 200 and 10,000 Hz). This could probably be reduced, if not overcome, by enrolling the ageing person with Down syndrome in regular 'resensitization' sessions to a large variety of intensities and sound frequencies; exercises aiming at restating and refining the discriminative capacities of the elderly regarding a variety of sounds characteristics of ordinary life situations, objects, and events.

Productive lexical support

Reduced word fluency and additional difficulties in retrieving less frequent verbal material is a characteristic of older people. This might be quite handicapping in some situations of communication, particularly outside of the protected settings. It should be possible to reduce this difficulty, or at least to keep it within socially acceptable limits, by regularly refreshing the functional lexical repertoires through systematic exercises of naming from pictorial material. Computers offer an almost infinite number of possibilities easy to adapt to the needs of every person with intellectual disability in maintenance training.

Receptive and productive language processing

There is evidence (cf. Maxim and Bryan, 1994 for a review) that the ability of the typical elderly to understand and produce combinatorial language (particularly longer and syntactically more complex sentences) differs from that of younger age groups. The ability to understand and produce complex language may deteriorate with age, as shown in experimental conditions. In typically ageing people, however, various strategies are used in life conditions in an often successful attempt to compensate for this relative decline. It is important to keep in mind that basic morphosyntax and the ability to coordinate the necessary semantic and grammatical processes remain largely unhampered in typical ageing. Only the more complex formal structures appear to cause problems in an important proportion of normal elderly people beyond the 60s and the early 70s.

Among the problematic formal structures in language comprehension of typically ageing people, one finds (expectedly as these structures are later mastered by typically developing children in language development) the double object construction (for example, 'he showed the lady the baby'), subordinate clauses headed by the adverbial temporal markers *before* and *after* (or corresponding ones), particularly when the order of the events referred to does not correspond to the enunciation order (for example, 'she sat down after she finished her cleaning'). In the same way, left-branching complex sentences (for example, 'because he felt uneasy, he left the room'; as opposed to 'he left the room because he felt uneasy') are increasingly difficult to understand by elderly people. The same is true for sentences with embedded clauses (for example, subject or object relatives of the following type: 'the man whom I spoke to was the group leader'; 'the man who spoke to me was the group leader').

Considering *language production*, the comparative age research points to an increase in performance errors, such as higher proportions of uncompleted sentences. The elderly need more time to process language for production. As a consequence, certain phenomena, such as filler expressions and phrases, appear more frequently as masking and time-gaining strategies. The elderly also tend to use fewer longer, complex sentences, and/or embedded clauses, confirming some organizational difficulty in language output.

There is no reason why ageing people with Down syndrome could or should escape this apparently common language-processing fate. However, for the those with Down syndrome, the matter gets potentially considerably more serious given that their final levels of morphosyntactic development are already considerably lower than normal. A decline in receptive and productive processing will unavoidably curtail most seriously their combinatiorial language ability. At present we do not have the data to specify the range of these problems. Assuming that they indeed manifest themselves with the intensity that could be feared, it would be most important to set up preventive maintenance grammatical activities with these people. The exact definition, scope, and contents must await precise empirical indication from research.

Discourse processing planning and monitoring

There are also clear indications that the typical older people have additional difficulties in processing longer discourse (stories, argumentative pieces, theoretical discourse, and so forth) and in planning and executing them swiftly. It seems likely that memory capacity limitations are involved to an important extent in these difficulties. Light and Albertson (1990), for example, found that elderly non-disabled adults could process textual inferences as well as younger ones when requested to do so within the constraints of their short-term memory. They had difficulty with larger spanning information because they either forgot some aspects crucial to extracting the inferences or had difficulty in reorganizing the textual material in working memory.

Discourse production may also become more problematic with increasing age. Stories that are told, for instance, may prove less cohesive (for example, Ulatowska, Cannito, Hayaski, and Fleming, 1985; Stine and Wingfield, 1990). Reasons for this state of affairs may involve multiple factors, such as sensory impairments, short-term memory limitations and difficulties in integrating expanded information.

Younger persons with Down syndrome typically have important difficulties in dealing receptively as well as productively with textual information, macrostructures and cohesion. It is conceivable that these difficulties could increase in later years. Preventive training could profitably concentrate on discourse macrostructures and cohesion maintaining strategies. Discourse macrostructures are default regulations applying to textual organization and particular to each type of discourse. Storytelling, for instance, implies a chronological sequence of steps of episodes (which may be short or extended). According to Halliday (1985), there are four ways by which textual cohesion is strengthened: reference, ellipsis, conjunction, and lexical continuity. *Reference* means that a participant or circumstantial element introduced at one place in text can be taken as a reference point for something that follows (for example, *The boy who looks after the sheep . . . he . . . him . . . he*). *Ellipsis:* a clause, part of a clause, or part of a nominal or verbal group may be presupposed at a subsequent place in the text. Either this element is omitted or it is replaced by a substitute element (for example, the *do* in *I will not wake him up for if I do . . .*). *Conjunction:* a clause or some longer portion of text may be related to what follows by one of a set of semantic relations and *lexical continuity* established by the choice of words. This may take the form of word repetition, the choice of a word that is related semantically to a previous one, or the presence of 'key words' – words having special significance for the meaning of the particular text.

Numerous language activities are easily imagined in order to bolster discourse planning and cohesion. Audiovisual autoscopy and role playing may be particularly useful in helping individuals with Down syndrome to realize better their textual limitations and contribute to maintaining or training better discursive functioning.

Speech and language therapy for the elderly, and particularly for those with Down syndrome, is a slowly developing specialty that will certainly require an evaluation of its effectiveness and demand adequate knowledge from the professionals, not to mention a much stronger research basis. The cost of providing continued support and maintenance training to ageing people with Down syndrome is no doubt significant. However, such programmes would certainly prove effective in keeping persons with Down syndrome better functioning for longer periods of time, therefore saving the cost of increased institutional care, as well as promoting continued wellbeing and reducing psychological stress.

Note

1 The first part of this chapter is based on Rondal and Comblain (2002) Language in aging persons with Down syndrome. Down Syndrome Research and Practice 8 (1): 1–9.

References

Appel J, Kertesz A, Fishman M (1982) A study of language functioning in Alzheimer's patients. Brain and Language 17: 73–91.

Aufray C, Jukel J (2001) Effets généraux et différentiels d'un programme d'entraînement multimodal chez la personne âgée. L'Année Psychologique 101: 65–89.

Baird P, Sadovnick A (1995) Life expectancy in Down syndrome. Lancet 2: 1354–6.

Berry P, Groenweg G, Gibson D, Brown R (1984) Mental development of adults with Down's syndrome. American Journal of Mental Deficiency 89: 252–6.

Bishop D, Byng S (1984) Accessing semantic comprehension: methodological considerations and a new clinical test. Cognitive Neuropsychology 1: 223–43.

Brion S, Plas J (1987). Etat actuel de l'approche histopathologique des démences. Psychologie Médicale 19: 1235–42.

Brown W (1985) Genetics of ageing. In M Janicki, H Wisniewski (eds) Aging and developmental disabilities: issues and approaches. Baltimore Md: Brookes, pp. 185–94.

Burt D, Loveland K, Chen Y-W, Chuang A, Lewis K, Cherry L (1995) Aging in adults with Down syndrome: report from a longitudinal study. American Journal of Mental Retardation 100: 262–70.

Campbell-Taylor I (1993) Communication impairments in Alzheimer disease and Down syndrome. In J Berg, H Karlinsky, and A Holland (eds) Alzheimer disease, Down syndrome and their relationship. New York: Oxford University Press, pp. 175–93.

Chapman R (1999) Language development in children and adolescents with Down syndrome. In J Miller, M Leddy, L Leavitt (eds) Improving the Communication of People with Down Syndrome. Baltimore Md: Brookes, pp. 41–60.

Chevrie-Müller V (1981) Epreuves pour l'examen du langage: batterie composite. Paris: Editions du Centre de Psychologie Appliquée.

Comblain A (1995) Batterie pour l'Evaluation de la morpho-syntaxe. Liège: Laboratoire de Psycholinguistique de l'Université de Liège (unpublished).

Comblain A (1996) Mémoire de travail et langage dans le syndrome de Down. Doctoral thesis in Psychology (Logopedics), Université de Liège, Belgium (unpublished).

Dani A, Pietrini P, Furey M, McIntosh A, Grady C, Horwitz B, Freo U, Alexander G, Shapiro M (1996) Brain cognition in metabolism in Down syndrome adults in association with development of dementia. NeuroReport 7: 2933–6.

Das J-P, Divis B, Alexander J, Parrila R, Naglieri J (1995) Cognitive decline due to ageing among persons with Down syndrome. Research in Developmental Disabilities 16: 461–78.

Deb S, De Silva N, Gemmel H, Besson J, Smith F, Ebmeier K (1992) Alzheimer's disease in adults with Down syndrome: The relationship between the regional cerebral blood flow equivalents and dementia. Acta Psychiatrica Scandinavia 86: 340–5.

Devenny D, Hill A, Patxot O, Silverman W, Wisniewski H (1992) Ageing in higher functioning adults with Down's syndrome an interim report in a longitudinal study. Journal of Intellectual Disability Research 36: 241–50.

Devenny D, Silverman W, Hill A, Jenkins E, Sersen E, Wisniewski H (1996) Normal ageing in adults with Down's syndrome: a longitudinal study. Journal of Intellectual Disability Research 40: 208–21.

Dupont A, Vaeth M, Videbech P (1986) Mortality and life expectancy of Down's syndrome in Denmark. Journal of Mental Deficiency Research 30: 111–20.

Florez J (2000) El envejecimiento de las personas con sindrome de Down. Revista Sindrome de Down 17: 16–24.

Fowler A (1990) Language abilities in children with Down's syndrome: evidence for a specific syntactic delay. In D Cicchetti, M Beeghly (eds) Children with Down Syndrome: A Developmental Perspective. New York: Cambridge University Press, pp. 302–28.

Frostig M, Maslow P, Lefever D, Whittlesy J (1963) The Marianne Frostig Developmental Test of Visual Perception. Palo Alto Calif: Counsulting Psychologist Press.

George M, Thewis B, Van der Linden M, Salmon E, Rondal JA (2001) Elaboration d'une batterie d'évaluation des fonctions cognitives de sujets âgés porteurs d'un syndrome de Down. Revue de Neuropsychologie 11(4): 549–79.

Halliday M (1985) An Introduction to Functional Grammar. London: Arnold.

Hart A (1988). Language and dementia: a review. Psychological Medicine 18: 99–112.

Hoffman J, Hamson M, Welsh K, Earl N, Raine S, Delong D, Coleman R (1996) Interpretation variability of 18FDG-positron emission tomography studies in dementia. Investigation in Radiology 31: 316–22.

Holland A, Oliver C (1996) Down's syndrome and the links with Alzheimer's disease. Journal of Neurology, Neurosurgery and Psychiatry 59(2): 111–14.

Jancar J, Jancar P (1996) Longevity in Down syndrome: a twelve year survey (1984–1995) Italian Journal of Intellectual Impairment 9: 27–30.

Jodar M (1992) Envejecimiento normal versus demencia de Alzheimer. Valor del lenguaje en el diagnostico differencial. Revista de Logopedia, Foniatria y Audiologia 12: 171–9.

Kempler D, Curtiss S, Jackson C (1987) Syntactic preservation in Alzheimer's disease. Journal of Speech and Hearing Research 30: 343–50.

Lenneberg E (1967) Biological Foundations of Language. New York: Wiley.

Light D, Albertson S (1990) Comprehension of pragmatic implications in young and older adults. In D Burke, L Light (eds) Language, Memory and Aging. Cambridge: Cambridge University Press, pp. 122–57.

Mann D (1992) The neuropathology of the amygdala in ageing and in dementia. In J Aggleton (ed.) The Amygdala: Neurobiological Aspects of Emotion, Memory, and Mental Dysfunction. New York: Wiley-Liss, pp. 575–93.

Martin A (1987) Representations of semantic and spatial knowledge in Alzheimer's patients: implications for models of preserved learning and amnesia. Journal of Clinical and Experimental Neuropsychology 9: 121–4.

Maxim J, Bryan K (1994) Language of the elderly: a clinical perspective. London: Whurr.

Murillo Ruiz B (1999) Estudio de la evolucion del lenguaje en la demencia Alzeimer. Barcelona: ISEP Editorial.

Pedrabissi R, Soresi S (1989) Adattamento dell'ABI con oggetti RM di diversa gravità ed eziologia. Trento, Italy: Erickson.

Pickut B, Saerens J, Marien P, Borggreve F, Goeman J, Vandevivere J, Vervaet A, Diercks R, De Keyn P (1997) Discrimination use of SPECT in frontal lobe-type dementia versus (senile) dementia of the Alzheimer's type. Journal of Nuclear Medicine 38: 929–34.

Prasher V (1996) Age-associated functional decline in adults with Down's syndrome. European Journal of Psychiatry 10: 129–35.

Ribes R, Sanuy J (2000) Declive cognitivo en memoria y lenguaje: indicadores del proceso de envejecimiento psicologico en la persona con sindrome de Down. Revista Sindrome de Down 17: 54–9.

Rondal JA (1995) Exceptional Language Development in Down Syndrome. Implications for the Cognition Language Relationship. New York: Cambridge University Press.

Rondal JA, Comblain A (1996) Language in adults with Down syndrome. Down Syndrome Research and Practice 4(1): 3–14.

Rondal JA, Comblain A (2002) Language in ageing persons with Down syndrome. Down Syndrome Research and Practice 8(1): 1–9.

Rondal JA, Edwards S (1997) Language in Mental Retardation. London: Whurr.

Royston M, Mann D, Pickering-Brown S, Owen F (1994) Apolipoprotein E., e2 allele promotes longevity and protects patients with Down's syndrome from dementia. Neuro Report 5: 2583–5.

Saviolo-Negrin N., Soresi S, Bacichetti C, Pozzan G, Trevisan E (1990) Observations on the visual perceptual abilities and adaptive behaviour in adults with Down syndrome. American Journal of Medical Genetics, Supplement 7: 309–13.

Schapiro M, Haxby J, Grady C (1992) Nature of mental retardation and dementia in Down syndrome: study with PET, CL, and neuropsychology. Neurobiology of Aging 13: 723–34.

Schapiro M, Haxby J, Grady C, Duara R, Schlageter N, White B, Moore A, Sunadaram M, Larson S, Rapoport S (1987) Decline in cerebral glucose utilization and cognitive function with ageing in Down's syndrome. Journal of Neurology, Neurosurgery, and Psychiatry 50: 766–74.

Strauss D, Eyman R (1996) Mortality of people with mental retardation in California with and without Down syndrome, 1986–1991. American Journal of Mental Retardation 100: 643–51.

Stine E, Wingfield A (1990) The assessment of qualitative age differences in discourse processing. In T Hess (ed.) Aging and cognition: knowledge, organization and utilization. Amsterdam: Elsevier, pp. 192–226.

Thompson S (1999) Examining dementia in Down's syndrome. Decline in social abilities in Down syndrome compared with other learning disabilities. Clinical Gerontologist 20: 23–44.

Ulatowska H, Cannito M, Hayashi M, Fleming S (1985) Language abilities in the elderly. The Aging Brain: Communication in the Elderly. London: Taylor & Francis, pp. 87–112.

Van Buggenhout G, Lukusa S, Trommelen J, De Bal C, Hamel B, Fryns J-P (2001) Etude pluridisciplinaire du syndrome de Down dans une population résidentielle d'arriérés mentaux d'âge avancé: Implications pour le suivi médical. Journal de la Trisomie 21(2): 7–13.

Vicari S, Nocentini U, Caltagirone C (1994) Neuropsychological diagnosis of ageing in adults with Down syndrome. Developmental Brain Dysfunction 7: 340–8.

Wilson B, Ivani-Chalian R (1995) Performance of adults with Down's syndrome on the Children's version of the Rivermead Behavioural Memory Test. British Journal of Clinical Psychology 34: 85–8.

Wisniewski H, Silverman W (1996) Alzheimer disease, neuropathology and dementia in Down syndrome. In JA Rondal, J Perera, L Nadel, A Comblain (eds) Down Syndrome: Psychological, Psychobiological and Socio-educational Perspectives. London: Whurr, pp. 43–52.

Wisniewski H, Silverman W (1999) Down syndrome and Alzheimer disease: variability in individual vulnerability. In JA Rondal, J Perera, L Nadel (eds) Down Syndrome. A Review of Current Knowledge. London: Whurr, pp. 178–94.

Ylieff M (2000a) Evaluation neuropsychologique de Françoise (document confidentiel). Liège, Université de Liège, Service de Psychologie de la Santé, Unité de Psychologie Clinique du Vieillissement, May.

Ylieff M (2000b). Personal communication with JA Rondal.

Zigman W, Schup N, Haaveman M, Silverman W (1997) The epidemiology of Alzheimer disease in intellectual disability: Results and recommendations from an international conference. Journal of Intellectual Disability Research 41: 76–80.

:lusion

SUE BUCKLEY, JEAN A RONDAL

The chapters in this book indicate that there is a great deal of relevant knowledge on the speech and language development of individuals with Down syndrome to guide the work of speech and language therapists, teachers and parents. The content of the chapters also justifies our argument for considering the modularity of the components of speech and language. It is clear that it is helpful to consider the literature on each component skill separately and to consider individual therapy targets for each.

It is important to note that the typical difficulties for children with Down syndrome vary in degree. Usually pragmatics and semantics are relative strengths over time whereas grammar and phonology are relative weaknesses. Working memory difficulties also contribute to weaknesses in discourse skills for teenagers and adults. Awareness of this profile is important in planning therapy and the semantic strengths explain why augmentative communication systems can be so helpful.

In addition, many individuals understand more than they can express – they have a gap between their comprehension of language and their expressive abilities and, therefore, separate targets may be needed for developing comprehension and expression.

It is clear that there is a growing knowledge base that has moved on from simply describing the characteristics of the speech and language of individuals with Down syndrome to beginning to give clear indications of some of the possible underlying causes, such as limited verbal short-term memory development, but there is still a need for much more research. In particular, there is a need for research studies that consider the interactive effects of specific difficulties in one domain on development in the others.

For example, little attention has been given to the effects of significant difficulties and delays in the development of speech-motor skills on the development of expressive language. The work reviewed in Chapter 4 hints at the connection as two of the studies it describes record an increase in mean length of utterance (MLU) as a result of targeting phonology. In addition to directly affecting what a child or adult can say, the speech-motor delays and the unintelligible speech are highly likely to distort the way others talk to the person. It is possible that the usual expansion of utterances to complete sentences that is provided by parents when children are at a two- or three-word stage of production may be distorted as the parent may have to repeat the child's utterance to check understanding before the conversation can proceed. There is a need for longitudinal research that takes account of the complexities of these possible interactive effects.

The authors of each chapter provide specific guidance for interventions, based on the evidence available from research on typical development and on development for individuals with Down syndrome. However, every author highlights the lack of evaluation of intervention. Very few interventions have been systematically evaluated. This is a difficult task and, again, it requires longitudinal studies. Such studies need to take account of the wide range of individual differences that exist between children with Down syndrome. Evaluations that present only group data are useful in that they may demonstrate the possibility of creating positive change, but the group data often conceal large individual differences – some individuals make large gains, some small gains and some may even lose rather than gain skills – when the overall effect is still a significant group gain. The reasons for the individual differences may be, in part, due to the characteristic difficulties of the person with Down syndrome, or the resources of their families or the school or day-care setting. Some interventions may work well with some individuals and not others or in some settings and not others.

This leads to a need for the research community to ensure that individual differences, and all the family, social and community factors that may influence outcomes, are documented and explored in research studies. It may also mean a shift towards encouraging speech and language therapists to document their work and publish more case studies. The collection of data through case studies can be systematized by developing protocols for data collection that can be shared, so that the same data are collected for each individual case. The authors are aware that practising speech and language therapists (and parents) have a wealth of knowledge and information that is never documented. If the research and professional practice communities could establish systematic ways of recording and sharing data, perhaps a shared store of information on children and adults could be established, as exists for data on typically developing children. This would lead to an increase in knowledge and it might also lead to the identification of important hypotheses for new experimental research.

A theme of this book has been the need to take a lifespan perspective. This has a number of implications. First, the authors wish to draw attention to the need for interventions to be age appropriate and to take account of the communication requirements of individuals within their environments. Second, they wish to identify the importance of offering intervention across the lifespan and to stress that some aspects of speech, language and communication skills improve into adult life. Here again, more research is needed as the chapters by Rondal and Jenkins on adults indicate how little objective information we have. Parents frequently comment on the continued improvement of spoken language in adult life into the thirties, but this has not been systematically documented. Does improvement represent the effects of practice and confidence on speech intelligibility and/or are there developments in expressive grammar? The appearance of improvement in expressive grammar observed by parents may be a result of improvement in speech-motor skills with practice, thus enabling the individual to express more complete sentences, rather than reflecting new grammatical learning.

This raises a third point with respect to age – are there indeed critical or optimal periods for components of the language system? Buckley, in her chapter on reading, has raised this issue by suggesting that the effects of reading instruction that begins before 3 years of age seem to be qualitatively and quantitatively different. She draws on deafness literature to support the view that the first five years are vitally important and that at this stage the brain is optimally ready to learn a first language. The implications of this view are that therapists and parents should focus great efforts on developing children's communication skills at this time, as it may not be possible to compensate later for progress lost at this time. This does not mean that children and adults do not progress after five years – steady progress is recorded until teenage years in all domains – but research with deaf individuals shows that gains made in the first five years convey a long-term advantage. The next issue in relation to critical periods is regarding grammatical and phonological progress. Is it possible to learn new grammar or to improve phonology after mid- to late teenage years? These are issues on which again we need systematic research, and at present there are opposing views.

Current evidence would lead the authors to advocate that early interventionists take seriously the importance of language learning in the first five years and do not miss the opportunity to encourage as much development as possible at this time, while also stressing that progress will be made by most children, throughout their childhood, in all domains. In late teenage and early adult life it is not yet clear what progress is possible and therefore therapy should still encourage development in all domains, while recognizing that development of grammar may be more difficult with age.

It is hoped that the contents of this book will encourage therapists to raise their expectations for individuals with Down syndrome and will increase the priority given to speech and language work with individuals from birth to adult life. The authors would be pleased to hear from anyone interested in their suggestion of establishing a systematically collected database of information on the speech, language and communication profiles of individuals with Down syndrome.

Appendix 1
Major acquisitions in morphosyntactic development[1]

JEAN A RONDAL

I. The acquisition of major semantic relations

The semantic relational basis of a given language (originating in general cognition) comprises a set of properties and relations between entities represented lexically in the language that are coded formally in the morphosyntax of this language. The semantic basis, therefore, is central for morphosyntactic development and functioning. Sentences are only rule-governed formalizations of networks of semantic relations. Understanding a sentence (linguistically) amounts to moving backward from its surface to the array of semantic relations and lexical meanings that may be plausibly supposed to have been at the starting point of the sentence construction process in the speaker's head, using relevant grammatical knowledge. Expressing a sentence involves the same operations but the other way around, moving from communication motivations and non-linguistic ideas on to semantic relations and their lexical and grammatical expression.

1.1. Two-word stage

At first, children use single words to communicate and then they begin to put two words together to convey more information, usually according to the following semantic relations. No exact grammatical sequential order or inflexional marking of the lexemes matters at this stage. What is important is the understanding and expression of lexicalized semantic relations.

- Possession (for example: 'mummy car').
- Location-position ('in box').
- Qualitative attribution ('blue ball').
- Temporal ('go now').
- Quantitative attribution ('two ball').

- Existence notice ('that biscuit').
- Non-existence, denial, rejection, disappearance ('no banana'; 'allgone juice').
- Recurrence ('more biscuit').
- Conjunction ('cup plate').
- Instrument ('with brush')
- Accompaniment ('with daddy').
- Ambient ('rain fall').
- Agent–action ('mummy push').
- Agent–object ('drink juice').
- Agent–object ('daddy shoe' as he puts his shoe on, for instance).

1.2. Three-word stage

Extending his or her two-word utterances, the child will gradually produce three keyword utterances modelled after the following major semantic relations (other combinations may be observed, however) either in declarative or yes–no interrogative form (a question form based on the intonation of the utterance).

- Agent–action–object (Daddy hit ball)
- Agent–action–locative (Mummy go store)
- Action–object–locative (Take shoe bathroom)
- Prepositional relation (car in box)
- Experiential utterance (Baby want biscuit)
- Phrase with modifier (Want more cheese).

Utterances with four or five words (and more) will then become possible by recombination of preceding structures.

2. Building up phrases

Phrases are the building blocks of sentences. They are formed of particular lexemes disposed in specific orders around a syntactic head. As a consequence, at this level of development, sequential ordering matters but not, instead, the appropriate use of morphological inflections for marking grammatical concord. The major phrases in the English language for my limited purpose here are: nominal, verbal, attributive, and prepositional. I shall leave aside the adverbial and the conjunction phrases (see Halliday, 1985, for example, for more details).

2.1. Phrases

Noun phrases (NPs) centre around a semantic core and syntactic head that may be either a common noun, a proper noun, or a personal pronoun; preceding or following the head, one may have one or several modifiers (for example, articles, qualifiers, quantifiers, classifiers, deictics).

- Article + common noun ('the ball'; 'a pencil').
- Article + qualifier + noun ('a red ball').
- Quantifier + noun ('two balls').
- Article + noun + classifier ('the house (of) the doggie').
- Deictic + noun ('my house'; 'that house').
- Linear combinations of preceding structures ('the little house (of) the doggie').

Verb phrases (VPs): They are constituted by a conjugated verb, as head of phrase, followed by one (or several) NPs.
- Verb + NP [(Mummy) cooks the meal].

Prepositional phrases (PPs) are composed of a preposition (head of phrase) followed by a NP.
- Prepositional + NP [(ball) under the car].

Attributive phrases (APs): They are preceded by an auxiliary verb and have an attribute (of the grammatical subject) as head, which may be accompanied by a modifier (e.g., adverb). Most of the time, the attribute is an adjective.
- Auxiliary-Be + AP + adjective [(The house) is red]
- Auxiliary-Be + AP + modifier + adjective [(The doggie) is all black]

2.2. Function words

As the examples in the first section above show, early combinatorial language is mostly deprived of function (or grammatical) words such as articles, pronouns, auxiliaries, and prepositions. The following steps in development will concern the comprehension and the production of these structures. This development is quite complex linguistically and cognitively and, as a consequence, is usually spread over a longer period of time even in the typically developing child.

Articles

The correct use of the articles 'the' and 'a' may be difficult because they are not stressed in normal talk and therefore identifying and processing them are more delicate operations. Strictly speaking, their contrastive use adds little to the meaning of the phrase, permitting only to distinguish between specific and non-specific reference.

Pronouns

Pronouns are also delicate structures, replacing nouns in discourse. Some are dialogic entities (for example, 'I', 'you', 'we', 'me') referring to the speaker or the person spoken to. Others (for example, 'they', 'it', 'them', 'their') refer to entities outside the dialogic context. For these third-person personal pronouns, co-reference with the noun replaced by the pronoun must be established for the sentence to be intelligible. Most often, co-reference is formally indicated by agreement in gender and number between pronoun and noun (for example, 'the little girl, she wore a red hat'). Pronominal co-reference takes some time to be mastered by typically developing children. It may be expected to cause a particular problem in comprehension and production for younger Down syndrome children.

Auxiliaries

In the same way as the articles, the auxiliary verbs such as 'is' and 'are', may be difficult because they are not usually stressed in talk and because they add little or no meaning to the sentence. They are mostly connecting structures. DS children often have difficult learning to use them in their language.

Prepositions

The most common prepositions are those related to spatial localization, temporal succession, instrumentation and accompaniment. Within spatial prepositions, the easiest to master are the topological ones, marking relations of vicinity (for example, 'in', 'on', 'under', 'next to'). The projective prepositions (e.g., above, below, ahead of, at the front, at the back, on the left, on the right) are more difficult (cognitively). The latter demand that some sort of rule-governed projection be made on the entities designed in order to decide what part of it is front, back, left, and so forth. Temporal prepositions (for example, 'before', 'after') require that at least some minimal time structuring be in place for appropriate use.

3. Marking number concord and possession within phrases

The use of /s/ on the end of a word to indicate a plural is a grammatical rule that is learned early in typical development. A number of words have irregular plurals (such as foot–feet, tooth–teeth). They have to be learned individually for there are no simple ways to tell them apart in advance from the words that form regular plurals.

The use of /'s/ following the end of a word to indicate possession (the so-called Saxon genitive) is also learned relatively early by typically developing children. It is preceded by possessive pronouns of first and second persons and occurs alongside the regular use of third person possessive ones.

4. Integrating phrases into basic sentences

Basic sentences (i.e., simple declarative affirmative actives) may be classified according to some of their most frequent structural compositions (full correct inflectional markings on verbs do not matter at this stage).

- NP–VP–NP (simple transitive structures, for example: 'The dog chases the cat.' 'The man drives his car.')
- NP–VP (simple intransitive structures, for example: 'The dog barks.' 'Baby sleeps.')
- NP–VP–NP–PP (more complex transitive structures, for example, 'The dog chases the cat in the yard.')
- NP–VP–PP (more complex intransitive structures, for example, 'The dog barks in the yard.')
- NP–Aux–Attribute (simple attributive structures, for example, 'The dog is big.' 'The man is tall.')
- Transitive or intransitive structures modified by an adverb (for example, 'The man drives his car fast.' 'The dog barks loudly.')

'Ing forms' (progressive forms) may be substituted for the non-progressive forms in some of the above combinatorial structures (for example, 'The dog is barking.' 'The man was driving his car fast.')

5. Different syntactic pragmatic types of sentences

Expressing the most basic functional types of sentences (declaring, negating, questioning) is, of course, of utmost importance in interpersonal communication. From quite early on, children understand and can use 'no' when they do not want something or to do something. However, the proper formulation of negative sentences comes substantially later. In so doing, a negative adverb has to be positioned within the sentence to perform the negating function, which additionally implies dealing properly with the auxiliary verb (for example, compare the following declarative and negative forms: 'The cat is awake.' 'It does not sleep.' 'The man drives his car.' 'He does not eat.' 'The dog is small.' 'It is not big.')

In a similar way, the typically developing child will display understanding of (unanalysed) question forms such as 'What's that?' 'Who's coming?' from quite early, and they will sometimes ask questions at the one-word stage by pointing or using something sounding like the interrogative word 'what?' However, the proper formulation of question sentences will come later. Two subtypes of questions may be distinguished: the 'yes–no' and the 'wh' questions. The first ones are based either on a particular intonation pattern (raising intonational level at the end of the sentence instead of lowering it as is normally the case for declarative sentences) – for example, 'John went there?' – or inverting the subject-verb order canonical for declarative sentences (for example, 'was John there?'). The 'wh' questions are constructed in such a way that a particular type of information is requested from the responder through the use of specific interrogative pronouns or adverbs. For example, a question such as 'who was there?' with an agent word, 'when did that happen?' with a time-referring word; 'what did you do?' with an object word or phrase, and so forth.

6. Morphological inflections on verbs

Inflectional markings of three (non-orthogonal) types are effectuated on main verbs and auxiliaries. They are concerned with the person and the number of the grammatical subject (of the verb) and with the temporal aspectual relationships holding for the sentence.

Person and number markings are made on main and auxiliary verbs using particular inflections (for example, 'I sleep'; 'she sleeps'; 'I am'; 'you are'; 'he is'; 'we are'; 'they are') and personal subject pronouns. The first two persons are dialogue forms and the third ones are exophoric (as explained above).

Basic temporal organization is made around tenses referring to past, present, and future events (and relationships between events) in relation to the locutor's situation in time. To form many tenses properly, an auxiliary verb is needed (for example, 'he will be going'; 'he has been there'). The past tense of verbs comes in two forms, regular and irregular. The regular form is the 'ed'-form (for example, jumped, pushed). The irregular forms are all different and as a consequence have to be learned individually (for example, 'slept', 'ran', 'made', 'came', 'had'). Irregular verbs are among the most frequently used entities in the English verbal system (actually, historically, this is the major reason why they have become irregular). A number of irregular past tense forms are often learned by typically developing children before they learn the 'ed' form. Development regarding this verbal structure is often 'U-shaped' – children learn the irregular (most frequent) past forms first, then learn some 'ed' forms; they then tend to generalize the 'ed rule' including (wrongly) to the irregular verbs (productions such as 'comed', 'eated', 'drinked', are observed at those times); eventually, they stabilize the correct dichotomy between regular and irregular verbal forms. Aspectual characteristics of the events referred to call for additional specifications justifying the existence of alternative 'tenses' in the grammar. Referring to past events, for instance, it is often the case that at least two aspectual tenses are distinguished. The so-called perfect tense referring to events that are completely finished and with no importance incidence on the locutory situation (for example 'he moved years ago') and, in opposition, the past tense or composite past form (for example 'he has moved'), which is used when the event referred to may be considered as having an incidence on the locutory situation. The imperfect tense will be used to refer to an event having lasted for some time in the past (for example, 'he was moving when we came').

7. More advanced formal structures

There are a number of more complex structures, either mono-propositional, such as the comparatives (for example, the series 'big, bigger, biggest'; or forms such as 'Daddy is taller than Mummy'), or bi-propositional (for example, 'John is taller than Bob but smaller than Robert').

More complex and later mastered sentence constructions by typically developing children include:

- 'X but not Y' sentences (for example, 'It is windy but not raining.')
- Sentences with a relative clause derived to the right of the main clause (for example, 'The man waited for a taxi that never came.') Also sentences with a relative clause embedded within the main clause (for example, 'The man whom I spoke to this morning was waiting for a taxi.') Embedded relatives are notoriously more difficult to process, everything else being equal, than right-derived ones. Relative pronouns may function either as subject or object of the main verb of the main clause (for example, 'The man who waited for a taxi wore a white hat.' 'The man I spoke to wore a white hat.' 'The man waited for a taxi that arrived after two hours.' 'The man took a taxi for which he never paid.')
- Reversible passive (for example, 'The black cat is chasing the white cat.') – as opposed to non-reversible (implausible reversible passive such as 'the operation was performed by the surgeon'); the former being more difficult to understand and correctly produced later by typically developing children.
- Sentences with circumstantial clauses (causal, consequential, and temporal ones, in particular). They may be produced with an order matching the order in which the (real or imaginary) events have happened, will happen, or are happening, or not (the latter being more difficult and being acquired later by typically developing children). Similarly, the sentences may follow the natural order cause–effect or consequence, or not (the latter again more difficult and acquired later). Contrast, for instance, the following formulations: 'The man had breakfast and left.' 'The man left after he had breakfast.' 'He was hit by the car and fell on the ground.' 'The man fell on the ground because he had been hit by the car.'

Note

1. Adapted, modified, and extended from Buckley 2000, and Rondal, 1986, 1997).

References

Buckley J (2000) Speech and language development for individuals with Down syndrome – An overview. Southsea, UK: Down Syndrome Educational Trust.

Halliday M (1985) An Introduction to Functional Grammar. London: Arnold.

Rondal JA (1986) Le développement du langage chez l'enfant trisomique 21. Manuel d'aide et d'intervention. Brussels: Mardaga.

Rondal JA (1997) Faire parler l'enfant retardé mental. Un anagramme d'intervention psycholinguistique. Brussels: Labor.

Appendix 2
Bilingual and multilingual issues[1]

JEAN A RONDAL

1. As the text on the programme leaflet of the Symposium correctly indicates: 'In a united Europe, knowing two or more languages will become a sine qua non for European citizens. Those who know only their mother tongue will see a considerable reduction in their communicative abilities. Such a situation could be considered a new form of illiteracy.' To this statement, one may add the obvious fact that intellectually disabled or not, a growing number of children are being educated at school through a second language with often little to no realistic language alternative: for example, children raised in Catalan homes and attending preschool and primary school in Castilian, or conversely; children raised in English and attending classes in Gaelic (two languages very different in many respects); children raised in Basque and taught in Castilian at school, or conversely (again two very different languages structurally). In such cases, and many others in Europe and in the World, sequential bilingualism is compelling. In many cases, for children with intellectual disabilities, familial situations of simultaneous bilingualism also exist (the two parents and/or grandparents being native speakers of different languages and practising them in conversing with other family members or other people).

2. Rightly then, a question asked more and more often by parents and other people concerned with intellectual disability, is whether it is reasonable or advisable to expose children with intellectual disabilities to developmental contexts and learning situations involving two languages and, if yes, what language benefits could be expected in the medium and longer term. I shall try to answer these two questions relying on indirect arguments and some anecdotal evidence because there is no research literature or systematic study of bilingualism in people with intellectual disabilities to inform decisions or recommendations.

3. Fifteen years ago, invited by Michel Paradis and Yvan Lebrun to express my prospective views on 'Bilingualism and mental handicap' as a chapter in a book on 'Early bilingualism and child development' (Rondal, 1984), I concluded from an analysis of language acquisition in children with intellectual disabilities that:

> It may be acceptable and perhaps useful to start bilingual education with *mildly* retarded children only a few years later than with normally developing children (say around a chronological age of 8 or 9 years). The situation, however, looks completely different when *moderately* and *severely* retarded individuals are taken into consideration. For these subjects, first-language acquisition is a strenuous, lengthy, and difficult endeavour, and it requires many years and much effort before they can attain a restricted productive and receptive capacity. So it would be extremely hazardous to risk systematic second-language training – let alone a complete immersion program – before late adolescence and without a favourable environment and maximum help from family and school . . . This is not to say that, if social circumstances make second-language learning necessary, a number of useful and functional vocabulary items and simple idiomatic structures could not be learned by moderately and severely retarded children . . . In this case, the only additional thing to teach the retarded subjects would be to discriminate between those situations that call for using items Xi . . . j from language X and those calling for the use of items Yi . . . j from language Y. This represents a simple case of discriminative learning of which most moderately and severely retarded subjects should be quite capable. (pp. 158–9; original emphasis)

4. Do we have reasons as of today to modify the preceding opinion? It would seem that we do indeed.

5. There is anecdotal evidence seemingly indicating (with all due methodological and interpretative caution) that a number of children and adults with intellectual disabilities exhibit some degree of bilingual competence (in the common sense of the term 'competence' and not the peculiar Chomskian one). Some of these children and adults are able to speak two, sometimes three languages, and a number of them, it would seem, are able to read and write to a functionally useful level in two languages. The levels of achievement seem to vary considerably between individuals.

Of course, the problem with anecdotal data is that their validity and reliability are difficult to establish. It is hard to know what they mean in terms of actual knowledge on the individuals' part. On such a basis, nothing can be proposed in general regarding children with intellectual disabilities, except perhaps rejecting the view that a bilingual situation at home or at school is necessarily going to be overwhelmingly difficult for these children.

Pursuing for a while the anecdotal observations of which I am aware, it can be added that the children and adults with intellectual disabilities who have developed some degree of bilingualism have had a variety of learning experiences. Some were raised in bilingual homes and have been exposed to two languages from birth (simultaneous bilingualism). They are reported as usually having more productive vocabulary and syntax in the language most frequently used in the family, while showing good comprehension of the other language.

Some other children and adults with intellectual disabilities have learned a second language outside the home as a result of going to school in a community that uses a different language from the child's first language (sequential bilingualism).

There are also cases of children with Down syndrome, born to profoundly deaf parents, who have become relatively fluent both in British Sign Language and English (simultaneous bimodal bilingualism). Buckley (1999), who reports the observations, signals that these children have met with difficulties in the grammatical aspects both of British Sign Language and English.

6. An issue bearing on the question of the capacity of children with intellectual disabilities for second language learning (L2) is that of the capacity of the same children for first language learning (L1). I am not dealing here with the problem – still very unclear and debated in the specialized literature – of the possible dependencies of L2 learning on L1 acquisition and mechanisms in sequential bilingualism (the question obviously is not fully relevant for simultaneous bilingualism).[2] Rather my purpose is to look for indications in the literature on language in intellectual disability that would be of particular help in answering my second question above, i.e., what to expect in terms of L2 acquisition judging from the difficulties encountered by people with intellectual disabilities in L1 development.

7. There exists an abundant literature on first language acquisition in children and adolescents with intellectual disabilities (see Rondal and Edwards, 1997, for a systematic review and analysis), particularly for what concerns individuals affected with Down syndrome, a genetic condition present in approximately one live birth out of 1,000 and due to a triplication of chromosome number 21, causing abnormal neurogenesis and a retardation level moderate to severe (modal intellectual quotient = 47).

Table A.1 lists the major language difficulties of typical individuals with Down syndrome.

From the indications in Table A.1, it can be hypothesized that L2 learning, if possible at all with most children with Down syndrome (which, optimistically considered, could be the case, at least for some degree of L2 learning), will meet with difficulties that correspond with those of L1 learning. This knowledge should therefore be made available to the teachers who would be involved in L2 programmes with mentally retarded individuals.

Table A.1. Major language problems in persons with Down syndrome.

Language component	Semiology
1. Sound articulation and auditory discrimination	*Articulatory and co-articulatory difficulties, particularly with the more delicate phonemes. Slow and sometimes incomplete maturation of phonemic discrimination.
2. Lexical semantics	Reduced lexicon both in number of lexemes and in semantic features within lexemes. * Poor organization of the mental lexicon, both semantically and pregrammatically.
3. Morphosyntax	Reduced length and formal complexity utterances. * Problems with inflexional morphology. * Problems with producing and understanding subordinated propositions and compound sentences.
4. Language pragmatics	Slowness of development in advanced pragmatic skills (e.g., topic contribution in conversation, interpersonal requests, monitoring verbal interactions with other people).
5. Discursive organization	* Insufficiently developed discourse macrostructures.

*The asterisks signal the most serious problems.

However, it is becoming clear that the etiology of intellectual disabilities (particularly for the genetic syndromes) has to be taken into account. The language profile associated with Down syndrome is in no way prototypical of language development and functioning in all people with intellectual disabilities.

Recent analyses of the language of individuals with intellectual disabilities affected with genetic conditions other than Down syndrome show that there exist important between-syndrome variations (Rondal and Comblain, 1999). This should be taken into account when considering L2 education or simultaneous bilingual exposure with children with these syndromes. Table A.2 summarizes comparative information on four syndromes associated with intellectual disabilities: Down syndrome, Williams syndrome (a congenital condition related to hemizygous deletions at chromosome 7q11.23, with an occurrence of 1 case in 10,000 live births), Fragile X syndrome (an X-linked disorder due to a null mutation of the FMR-1 gene at Xq27.3, that is passed on through generations with a prevalence close to 0.25 per 1,000 males; it is less frequent in females), and Prader-Willi syndrome (the majority of cases being associated with deletions in the q11-13 region of chromosome 15 from paternal origin; the incidence is one case in approximately 20,000 live births). Many more specific syndromes are awaiting systematic investigation (Shprintzen, 1997).

Table A.2. Feature distribution in four mental retardation syndromes.

	Syndromes			
Language aspect	Down	Williams	Fragile X (affected males)	Prader-Willi
Phonetico-phonological	— —	+ +	— —	— —
Lexical	—	+	+	—
Morpho-syntactic	— —	+	—	—
Pragmatic	+	— —	— —	—
Discursive	— —	+	—	?

Key: +(+): relative strength; —(—): relative weakness; ?: absent or insufficent data.

It is worth adding that the between-syndrome variability has little to do with psychometric level. The levels and general cognitive abilities are roughly the same in the four syndromes documented (spanning from moderate to lower mild intellectual disability). Cognitive variables are not good predictors of development when it comes to the phonological and the morphosyntactic components of language, as I have shown elsewhere taking advantage of pathological cases and analyses (Rondal, 1995). In the genetic syndromes leading to intellectual disability it is becoming clear that the language developmental and functional characteristics of the syndromes are related to particulars of the neurogenesis (in the specialized language areas of the brain). For example, the brains of individuals with Down syndrome and Williams syndrome are morphologically different (Jernigan, Bellugi, Sowell, Doherty and Hesselink, 1993) in ways relevant to the language problems in each syndrome.

As indicated in Table A.2, the expectations one may have regarding L2 learning, either simultaneously or sequentially, in individuals with intellectual disabilities will vary substantially from one syndrome to the other. Extrapolating from L1 development, it is likely that individuals with Williams syndrome would demonstrate better L2 learning, particularly in the phonological, lexical, and productive morphosyntactic aspects, while experiencing serious pragmatic and communicative difficulties.

8. Substantial individual variations also exist within intellectual disability syndromes in L1 development. So-called exceptional cases of (first) language development in individuals with intellectual disabilities have been

documented (cf. Rondal, 1995, 1998; Rondal and Edwards, 1997; Rondal and Comblain, 1999; for reviews and analyses). Exceptional language in this context refers to levels of functioning not usually found in persons with moderate and severe intellectual disabilities although they are the norms for typically developing people. In most of the exceptional case studies so far, the language aspects most developed are phonology and receptive and productive morpho-syntax. Lexical development may also be particularly favourable in some cases.

Two cases of language-exceptional individuals with intellectual disabilities with a multilingual ability are relevant to my analysis. Vallar and Papagno (1993) have documented the case of an Italian girl with Down syndrome (standard trisomy 21). FF (the girl) was aged 23 at the time of the study and she had an IQ score of 71 points. She exhibited good acquisition of Italian (her maternal tongue) and to a lesser degree of English and French vocabularies and expressive morpho-syntax. The extent of her receptive ability in either language was not systematically evaluated. She showed correct articulation in the three languages, with occasional stuttering-like episodes. Up to the age of 6, FF lived in a NATO military base in Belgium where her father served as an officer. She practised her English with her sister-in-law who was British. According to Vallar and Papagno's report (1993), FF was able to hold a conversation with an English speaker, also on the phone, and to follow an English TV programme or movie. Her French was less fluent but, at the time of the study, she was practising it by herself using recorded tapes. She lived with her parents and she was working full time in an Italian advertising agency.

O'Connor and Hermelin (1991) and subsequently Smith and Tsimpli (1995) have reported on the provocative case of Christopher, a young adult with intellectual disability – etiology unknown; hydrocephaly had been offered as a diagnosis at some point – (25 to 29 years at the time of the studies) with an IQ of 67 but at a preoperational level on Piagetian scales.

Christopher has a mastery of English considered to be within the normal range, including the ability to detect morpho-syntactic violations (grammaticality judgements). Amazingly, he shows a good level of ability in translating in English from 13 languages (encompassing several families of languages): French, German, Spanish, Danish, Dutch, Finnish, Russian, Greek, Hindi, Norwegian, Polish, Portuguese, and Welsh. According to neurological reports, Christopher has severe impairment of his motor coordination, amounting to apraxia. He is also reported to have a minor speech defect. By 3 years chronological age, Christopher had begun to display his lifelong fascination with language, including early evidence of reading ability (having more to do with the forms than the contents). His interest in foreign languages began around 6 to 7 years of age. Christopher's lexical ability, for the languages he has been most exposed to, is impressive. On the Peabody Picture Vocabulary Test (PPVT), he scored at 121 in English, 114 in German, 110 in French, and 89 in

Spanish (the normal population mean for the PPVT is 100, standard deviation 15). For other languages (for example, Hindi), however, Christopher's abilities are rudimentary.

Analysing Ln abilities in Christopher, one can derive the following hierarchy: lexicon – inflexional morphology – syntax. His greatest strengths lie in learning the new words in a foreign language; than in pulling out morphological paradigms to deal with inflexional variants of those words. Syntax is often much less appropriate. He makes syntactic errors in translating sentences and paragraphs. In particular, he shows transfer from English to his subsequent languages in all aspects of syntax. Christopher resists word orders that are incompatible with the English dominant SVO pattern (subject–verb–object).

In conclusion, there are good reasons to suppose that Christopher's Ln abilities are lexically based overall and that the farther one moves from the lexicon along the continuum indicated above, the less able he is.

9. Speculating from the observations presented in what precedes, one can propose the following four points.

9.1. Learning foreign languages seems to be within the capacities of at least some children with intellectual disabilities (not only the more mildly affected ones). At the present stage, it is not possible, for lack of data, to specify what 'some' may mean in the sentence above (in other words, to which proportion of individuals with intellectual disabilities it applies, if not to all of them).

9.2. As in L1, important between-syndrome differences are to be expected in L2 learning.

9.3. As in L1 again, significant individual differences are to be expected in L2 learning.

9.4. It may be predicted that individuals with intellectual disabilities will meet with corresponding difficulties regarding the various language components and exhibit corresponding developmental delays in L2 as in L1 learning. Known problems in L1 development in the various genetic syndromes, therefore, are of interest in preparing to meet L2 difficulties. Of course, research should be promoted to test the above predictions and supply systematic data relevant to simultaneous and sequential bilingual learning in children and adolescents with intellectual disabilities. These data should bear on the various language components (phonology, lexicon, inflexional morphology and syntax, discourse, and pragmatic regulations).

10. Notwithstanding, there is a need for experimental bilingual language programmes for children and adolescents with intellectual disabilities to

be implemented in school settings. Special schools or classes, probably, would be well suited for this kind of applied research action and pedagogical innovation. Existing studies of this type are virtually non-existing to the best of my knowledge.

Reviewing the scarce pedagogical literature, I came across the summary of a study conducted in Kiev (Ukraine) (Vavina and Kovalchuk, 1986).[3] The majority of their children with intellectual disabilities (296 male and female Ukrainian children) demonstrated correct perception of speech, understanding of the sense of conversational replies, correct construction of utterances, and the ability to participate in a conversation in the initial stages of Russian-language instruction. But no information was supplied concerning the ages of the children, the type of intellectual disabilities, and the pedagogical techniques put to use.

There is a beginning literature, particularly in the USA, on multicultural and bilingual or multilingual special education (for example, Deutsch Smith and Luckasson, 1995). It aims at increasing the teachers' and the school administrators' awareness regarding the specific cultural and language needs of non-English-American children with intellectual disabilities raised in American public schools. In this literature, mention is made of the necessity for the teachers and the schools to rely more on what is labelled a 'mediational strategy'. In order to be effective for students with intellectual disabilities and limited English proficiency (the same is true for typically developing students), the following measures are suggested:

- use both English and the students' native language for instructional purpose
- integrate English language development with instruction in the content areas, and
- use information from the students' native cultures to enhance instruction.

These common-sense indications have little chance of being successful, however, if they are not backed by teachers' training and research in order to define what the specific language needs of the students with intellectual disabilities are in special or integrated school settings and daily classroom situations.

Based on current, admittedly scarce, knowledge of the capacities of students with intellectual disabilities for foreign language learning, what can one recommend in order to enhance L2 acquisition in these individuals, no matter how partial and incomplete it may remain?

The following four suggestions may be made.

10.1. Insist that systematic L2 exposure and/or training, in graduated immersion programmes or otherwise, be postponed for a few years (the precise delay remaining to be established from future relevant developmental data). Many immersion programmes for typically developing children start at around 4 years of age. These ages are generally considered to correspond to the period when typically developing children have learned enough of their maternal tongue to have it stabilized regarding the various basic receptive and productive aspects (phonology, lexicon, and morphosyntax). Adapting to the child with moderate or severe intellectual disability, one is speaking of roughly 6 or 7 years of age. What I am talking about is systematic L2 learning, not occasional or limited functional exposure. The thing that matters, in my view, is limiting L2 influence as long as some strong basis in L1 is not established, which, as is known, takes much more time in children with intellectual disabilities than in typically developing children. Acting otherwise could put the child with intellectual disability at great risk of having his/her first language acquisition process additionally retarded or disturbed.

10.2. In familial bilingual situations, one should try as much as possible to select the language of the school and community to be privileged as the basic language for daily use and therapy (not excluding the other familial tongue, however).[4] Later, when this selected L1 is stabilized to a sufficient extent, L2 exposure may be augmented with fewer risks of putting L1 development at risk.

10.3. Of course, L2 learning (even more than L1) will have to be functionally oriented in individuals with moderate and severe intellectual disabilities.

10.4. In individuals with intellectual disabilities, L2 learning will extend 'naturally' over longer periods of time than in typically developing people for results that generally will not match those of non-disabled individuals. Beyond childhood and early adolescence, extrapolating from L1 development again (cf. Rondal and Edwards, 1995), it is likely that the cost/benefit ratio in some aspects of L2 learning (particularly articulation, co-articulation, phoneme discrimination, and morphosyntax) will be less favourable. However, important learning benefits would still be expected regarding lexical and language pragmatic aspects.

Notes

1. Reproduced with permission from Saggi di Neurologia (2000) 16(1): 51–7; text of an invited Conference to the Symposium: 'Multilingual Education in Primary School in Europe', Istituto Eugeneo Medea, Udine, Italy, December 1999.
2. Much speculation has been offered in the recent (and less recent) literature, for example, in order to explain L2 learning's supposedly constant inferiority with regard to (NR) people's competence in L1, in

terms of theories involving the language properties described by universal grammar (UG) (for example, Smith and Tsimpli, 1995; cf. Epstein, Flynn and Martohardjono, plus commentaries, 1996, for a review and discussion). Such an approach presupposes, of course, that one accepts the UG concept as a valid one for explaining language learning, which certainly is controversial (cf., for example, Elman, Bates, Johnson, Karmiloff-Smith, Parisi and Plunkett, 1996).

3. Despite my efforts, I could not obtain either the Russian version of the paper or any commentary from the authors whom I tried to contact personally.

4. It would be rather cruel – and this is not my proposal – to tell parents or grandparents that they cannot communicate at all with a child in their first language.

References

Buckley S (1999) Bilingual children with Down's syndrome. Down syndrome: News and update 1: 29–30.

Deutsch Smith D, Luckasson R (1995) Multicultural and bilingual special education. In Introduction to special education. Boston Mass: Allyn & Bacon, pp. 39–77.

Elman J, Bates E, Johnson M, Karmiloff-Smith A, Parisi D, Plunkett K (1996) Rethinking innateness: a connectionist perspective on development. Cambridge Mass: MIT Press.

Epstein S, Flynn S, Martohardjono G, and commentaries (1996) Second language acquisition: theoretical and experimental issues in contemporary research. Behavioral and Brain Sciences 19: 677–758.

Jernigan T, Bellugi U, Sowell E, Doherty S, Hesselink J (1993) Cerebral morphologic distinctions between Williams and Down's syndromes. Archives of Neurology 50, 186–91.

O'Connor N, Hermelin B (1991) A specific linguistic ability. American Journal on Mental Retardation 95: 673–80.

Rondal JA (1984) Bilingualism and mental handicap. Some programmatic views. In M Paradis, Y Lebrun (eds) Early Bilingualism and Child Development. Lisse, Holland: Swets & Zeitlinger, pp. 135–59.

Rondal JA (1995) Exceptional language development in Down syndrome. Implications for the cognition–language relationship. New York: Cambridge University Press.

Rondal JA (1998) Cases of exceptional language in mental retardation and Down syndrome: explanatory perspectives. Down Syndrome Research and Practice 5(1): 1–15.

Rondal JA (2001) Language in mental retardation: individual and syndromic differences, and neurogenic variation. Swiss Journal of Psychology 60: 161–78.

Rondal JA, Comblain A (1999) Current perspectives on genetic dysphasias. Journal of Neurolinguistics 12: 181–212.

Rondal JA, Edwards S (1997) Language in Mental Retardation. London: Whurr.

Shprintzen R (1997) Genetic Syndromes and Communication Disorders. San Diego Calif: Singular.

Smith N, Tsimpli I (1995) The mind of a savant. Language Learning and Modularity. Oxford: Blackwell.

Vallar G, Papagno C (1993) Preserved vocabulary acquisition in Down's syndrome. The role of phonological short-term memory. Cortex 14: 89–101.

Vavina L, Kovalchuk V (1986) Characteristics of dialogic communication of mentally retarded schoolchildren under the conditions of Ukrainian–Russian bilingualism. Defektologia 4: 9–14.

Index

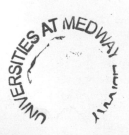